ESSENTIALS for PSYCHOPHARMACOLOGY FOR NURSE PRACTITIONERS

Deana Shevit Goldin, PhD, DNP, APRN, FNP-BC, PMHNP-BC, is a clinical associate professor at the Nicole Wertheim College of Nursing & Health Sciences, Florida International University. She is a nationally certified family and psychiatric mental health nurse practitioner and a fellow of the Integrative Psychiatry Institute. Dr. Goldin graduated from the University of Miami, Nova Southeastern University, Johns Hopkins University, and the Integrative Psychiatry Institute. Dr. Goldin has a broad background in healthcare with specific training in family practice and mental health across the life span, and works with diverse populations. Her practice experiences led to her observation that numerous clinical problems she encountered had significant psychological components; therefore, Dr. Goldin has published numerous articles focusing on uncommon and subtle psychiatric conditions that could easily be overlooked in primary-care settings. Through her assessments, she has become a leader in raising awareness and educating clinicians on the critical need to identify, manage, and appropriately recognize mental health disorders in primary-care settings.

ESSENTIALS for PSYCHOPHARMACOLOGY FOR NURSE PRACTITIONERS

Deana Shevit Goldin, PhD, DNP, APRN, FNP-BC, PMHNP-BC

SPRINGER PUBLISHING

Springer Publishing Company, LLC
11 West 42nd Street, New York, NY 10036
www.springerpub.com
connect.springerpub.com/

Acquisitions Editor: John Zaphyr
Compositor: Transforma

ISBN: 978-0-8261-8453-5

Printed by LSI

The *Essentials* series was published in the United States of America as the *Fast Facts* series.

I am forever grateful to be Andrew's mom.

Contents

Part IV ANSWERS TO REVIEW QUESTIONS

Preface

This book is intended for clinical healthcare providers, including physicians, nurses, advanced practice nurses, and other healthcare clinicians who need a practice guide, test review, or clinical resource guide that is easy to access and use. This book serves as a clinical guide to assist clinicians in prescribing psychotropic medications to address mental health conditions. This book can be used to assist clinicians to understand the key aspects of psychopharmacology.

Essentials for Psychopharmacology for Nurse Practitioners is the first practical guide for novice and experienced nurse practitioners for explaining and choosing appropriate psychiatric medications. This clinical reference is ideal for students and all clinically oriented healthcare professionals since it provides concise, bulleted-style text for easy access to pertinent information. This book offers readers a broad understanding of the key aspects of psychotropic medications used in general psychiatry and primary-care settings, and includes strategies to ease medication decision-making and evidence-based best practices for selecting and managing psychotropic medications.

Part I of this practical guide begins with an overview of general pharmacological principles and a brief overview of neurotransmitters, and covers the rationale for medication use and the risks and benefits of the major classes of psychotropic medications.

Part II includes medications across drug classes that are divided by age population and includes practice management strategies, safety considerations, drug interactions, identification of side effects and adverse reactions, basic laboratory test recommendations, treatment options, and self-management strategies.

Part III ends with important concepts for patient and/or caregiver education and advocacy.

Every chapter begins with learning objectives. Tables and "Essentials" boxes highlight important factors, adding further information for a fuller understanding of each topic. Each chapter includes references, website resources, practice questions, and further reading recommendations specific to the chapter topic for those interested in delving deeper. Answers to practice questions appear in Chapter 13.

This text is an evidence-based, user-friendly resource that can support clinicians to better understand, prescribe, monitor, assess, educate, and advocate for patients who are prescribed psychotropic medications, help promote safe patient encounters, and foster optimal patient outcomes.

Acknowledgments

No book is ever written in isolation, but rather is done with the consultation of pivotal experts. With that, I would like to sincerely acknowledge the editors at Springer Publishing for your professional guidance in facilitating the compilation of this book. To Dr. Maria Del Sol and Elizabeth Tapanes, thank you for your trust. To my husband, Keith, your voice is my favorite sound. To my son, your smile is my favorite sight and your laughter is my favorite music. To my mom, who is forever optimistic and sees the possibilities.

I

Introduction to Psychopharmacology

1

The Psychiatric Interview

Psychiatric mental health nurse practitioners (PMHNPs) apply a holistic and patient-centered approach to diminish mental distress and help mental health sufferers set attainable goals and have hope for the future. Using theoretically grounded methods, PMHNPs are trained experts in the evaluation and treatment of patients with disordered feelings, thoughts, and behaviors. Structured interviews, semistructured interviews, and questionnaires have become the gold standard for diagnostic interviewing for psychiatric mental health assessments. The goal of this chapter is to offer knowledge and skills required to conduct a mental health evaluation across populations.

In this chapter you will learn:

1. The purpose of the psychiatric interview
2. How to organize the initial psychiatric interview
3. How to assess for common psychiatric disorders
4. The purpose of the mental status exam
5. How to identify psychiatric emergencies

THE PSYCHIATRIC INTERVIEW AND ASSESSMENT

The purpose of a psychiatric interview is to establish rapport, develop a therapeutic relationship, and elicit a patient's personal narrative so as to collect, organize, and formulate an accurate diagnosis and treatment plan (American Psychiatric Association [APA], 2016). The PMHNP uses open-ended and closed-ended questioning and active listening techniques to ascertain the presence of particular symptoms and understand the patient.

Aims of the interview include (a) discovering the chief complaint(s); (b) reviewing the patient's history of the present illness; (c) reviewing the patient's mood, thought content and processes, and cognition; and (d) constructing a description of the patient's appearance, functionality, and reality. Psychiatric interviews provide an actionable psychopathologic format to derive a diagnostic classification for clinical decision-making (APA, 2016).

The primary tools used to evaluate and diagnose patients are the psychiatric interview and the mental status exam (MSE); however, history-taking and cognitive and behavioral assessments using screening tools and other evaluations are also used to aid clinicians in distinguishing between typical and atypical functioning and behaviors across a continuum. Essentially, the interview provides a method to assess a patient's anomalies of experiences, beliefs, expressions, and behaviors (Nordgaard et al., 2013).

There is not a "one size fits all" approach to the initial psychiatric assessment; for example, information gathering from additional sources such as family members, caregivers, friends, teachers, police officers, or healthcare providers may be required. This information may be included in the initial assessment; however, it may occur at a later time. If collateral information is necessary, it is important to explain why the information may be helpful to the patient and obtain written permission for the contact.

PRIMARY AIMS FOR THE PSYCHIATRIC INTERVIEW

The primary aims of a psychiatric interview are to describe a patient's complaints, appearance, experience(s), or existence; collect objective clinical data in an actionable psychopathologic layout for shared diagnostic classification; and guide treatment and clinical decisions.

GENERAL ASSESSMENT FOR COMMON PSYCHIATRIC DISORDERS

PMHNPs are expected to observe the significant positive and negative findings throughout the interview and document these findings into a particular format called the MSE (see Table 1.1). The MSE is the psychologic equivalent of the physical exam. It is a reliable and systematic approach to assess objective data of cognitive and behavioral functioning and subjective descriptions given from the patient. The purpose of the MSE is to provide a picture of the patient or a "snapshot" at a point in time. It is useful for the evaluation and diagnosis of a disorder and to appraise management and treatment responses (Table 1.2).

Like other assessment screenings in clinical practice, the MSE may have limitations and may be less sensitive to subtle cognitive impairments. Underlying medical conditions can elicit false-negative scores for patients who use alternative methods of coping to bypass their impairment. The MSE is also subject to the interviewer's skill, expertise, training, and interpretive bias, all of which can influence MSE assessment accuracy.

Table 1.1

Primary Aims for the Psychiatric Interview

Primary Aim	Steps
Identify patient and informant(s)	
Establish rapport	▪ Identify chief complaint ▪ Identify symptoms ▪ Allow patients time to tell their narrative
Elicit explicit information	▪ History of the present problem ▪ Precipitating factors ▪ Developmental history ▪ Allergies ▪ Medications (current and past) ▪ Past medical history ▪ Past psychiatric history ▪ Family background and medical/psychiatric history ▪ Social history and behavior patterns ▪ MSE ▪ General physical and neurologic exam ▪ Safety assessment
Manage the patient	▪ Form a diagnostic impression ▪ Review management and treatment recommendations ▪ Ask about unanswered questions or concerns

MSE, mental status exam

Table 1.2

Domains of the MSE

Appearance	Age; facial features; posture; grooming; weight; physical abnormalities
Behavior	Eye contact; alertness; cooperativeness; gait; movements; agitation
Speech	Rate; rhythm; volume; content
Mood	The patient's internal emotional state; personal internal experience; answer to the question "How are you feeling right now?"
Affect	Observable emotional state; external emotional expression
Thought Process	Flow of thoughts; associations of thoughts
Thought Content	Specific ideas and beliefs; perceptual disturbances
Cognition	Level of consciousness; general level of intellectual ability; memory; attention; general knowledge; executive functioning
Insight/ Judgement	Ability to understand one's own situation and ability make decisions to protect self and others

MSE, mental status exam

Essential Facts

Sensitivity and Specificity

- *Sensitivity* refers to those who have a disease or test positive; it represents or the true positive rate.
- *Specificity* refers to those who do not have the disease or who test negative; it represents the true negative rate.

Essential Facts

To accurately assess the MSE, remember to do the following:

- Collect information on the patient's education, culture, religion, worldview, and other social factors. For example, education level, insight, and judgment are fundamentally subjective, and personal beliefs may influence a patient's response.
- Ascertain the patient's norms; for example, some individuals always talk fast.

THE THERAPEUTIC ALLIANCE

The therapeutic alliance is a collaborative partnership between the patient and the provider. A therapeutic alliance occurs when the patient and provider are jointly engaged in purposive work centered around the patient's needs, goals, and desires (Allen et al., 2017). Every encounter with the patient can have therapeutic potential when providers use empathetic and deliberate dialogue. Characteristics of a therapeutic relationship include trust, acceptance, genuineness, empathy, respect, interpersonal authenticity, and maintenance of professional boundaries (Johnson & Vanderhoef, 2016). The therapeutic relationship includes three distinct phases, as outlined in Table 1.3.

Essential Facts

A strong alliance built on trust and respect has been shown to empower patients, decrease symptomatology, and promote positive treatment outcomes (McLeod et al., 2016). It includes the following:

- Building a therapeutic relationship
- Consistency
- Positive regard
- Attunement
- Attention to nonverbal cues
- Empathy

(*continued*)

Essential Facts (*continued*)

- Eye contact
- Educate and keep patient informed
- Use of developmentally appropriate language (i.e., consider other methods for nonverbal patients)

EVALUATION FOR PHYSICAL COMORBIDITIES

The considerable overlap in symptomatology between mental health disorders and physical disease processes complicates the clinical picture in the mental health arena. Unrecognized and untreated physical disorders have the potential to burden and negatively impact the care continuum.

It is important for clinicians to inquire about the patient's last comprehensive physical examination that included lab testing. Consider past and present core symptoms with attention to patterns and problem areas in the body, brain, and environment domains. PMHNPs are well equipped to detect underlying medical problems, distinguish normal versus abnormal symptoms, and identify when referrals are warranted. Consider using

Table 1.3

Phases of Therapeutic Relationship

Phase	Characteristics
Orientation Phase ▪ The introductory phase, which marks the start of the relationship and determines roles	▪ Relationship parameters are established, contracting (confidentiality, meeting length and time) ▪ Diagnostic evaluation ▪ Immediate concerns addressed ▪ Establish goals ▪ Key principles: effective communication, trust, and honesty
Working Phase ▪ The working phase of the relationship	▪ Data collection ▪ Issues and challenges are identified, problem-solving skills ▪ Exploration and identification of thoughts and ideas, explore view of self and others ▪ Continual assessment and identification of new problems ▪ Validation of thoughts and support positive change ▪ Measure outcomes and reprioritize aims; adjust management accordingly
Termination Phase ▪ The final phase of the relationship	▪ Appraise progress ▪ Reflect on accomplishments ▪ Promote self-management strategies ▪ Communicate feelings related to termination of relationship ▪ Disengage and refer if indicated ▪ Set parameters for further communication

screening or rating scales when patients are experiencing substance comorbidities such as substance misuse.

Clinicians should screen for both psychiatric and nonpsychiatric conditions. Initial lab testing to identify possible organic causes of illness includes (a) complete blood count (CBC); (b) chemistry panel; (c) hepatic panel; (d) thyroid labs; (e) vitamin D, B_{12}, and folate; (f) urine drug toxicology screen; (g) syphilis screening; (h) HIV screen; and (i) adrenal fatigue. Clinicians identify any abnormal neurologic findings and determine if brain imaging or a referral to a specialist is warranted.

Clinicians should assess the following environmental and lifestyle factors when screening for psychiatric and nonpsychiatric conditions:

- Attachments (insecure, disorganized, avoidant, ambivalent)
- Exercise
- Isolation
- Maladaptive behaviors
- Nutrition and diet, gluten sensitivity/allergy
- Relationship patterns
- Sexuality
- Sleep hygiene, insomnia, sleep apnea

Clinicians should also assess other considerations, such as trauma, singular traumatic events, complex trauma, disassociation, stressors and functioning, family, situational crises, employment, and relationships.

Essential Facts

Additional Screenings Specific to Children/Adolescents/Young Adults

- Development milestones assessment
- Lead screening
- Vision/hearing
- Sexually transmitted infections if suspected abuse or sexually active
- Thyroid disease
- Multiple sclerosis or other brain lesions
- Infection
- Dehydration
- Nutritional deficiencies
- Sexual activity and interest
- History of a head injury
- Sleep patterns

Essential Facts

Additional Screenings Specific to Older Adults

- Cancer screening exams (mammogram/colonoscopy/prostate exam)
- Lymph node exam

(*continued*)

Essential Facts (*continued*)

- New onset of cognitive deficits when older than 45 years of age
- Vision/hearing
- History of a head injury
- Sexually transmitted infections
- Thyroid disease
- Dehydration
- Infection
- Delirium
- Dementia
- Nutritional deficiencies
- Sexual activity and interest
- Sleep patterns

Essential Facts

- At birth, the average baby's brain is about a quarter of the size of the average adult brain and doubles in size in the first year. By age 3, the brain is about 80% of the adult size and nearly full grown by the age of 5 (Stiles & Jernigan, 2010).
- Childhood psychopathology requires a deep understanding of the complex interplay between neurobiologic, developmental, and environmental factors.

PUTTING IT ALL TOGETHER TO FORMULATE A DIAGNOSIS

Diagnoses are used in psychiatry to describe a syndrome or a cluster of both observable and reported symptomology (phenomenology) that co-occur and describe the patient's state. The *Diagnostic and Statistical Manual of Mental Disorders (DSM)* and *International Classification of Disease (ICD)* provide clinicians with a standardized diagnostic nomenclature that uses a descriptive and scientific algorithmic and categorial method toward psychopathology (Aboraya et al., 2016). The *DSM-5* (APA, 2013) serves as a guide to ensure diagnostic accuracy and has improved diagnostic reliability; however, increasing the validity of the *DSM-5* remains challenging (APA, 2016).

Essential Facts

Reliability and Validity

Reliability refers to the consistency of a measure (diagnosis); for example, a patient presenting with distinct symptoms would receive the same diagnosis if evaluated by different clinicians.

(*continued*)

Essential Facts (*continued*)

Validity is the extent to which the measure (diagnostic criteria) represents the variable (syndrome) it is intended to characterize; for example, clinicians who are determining validity consider whether the diagnosis represents the patient's actual symptomology or condition.

The use of labels (diagnosis) has the potential to be harmful and stigmatizing; however, in psychiatry, diagnoses are used to facilitate communication among clinicians and nonclinicians, and to facilitate interprofessional communication. Diagnoses also help support and gauge treatment outcomes (prognosis), measure incidence and prevalence of populations, identify population needs and other public health efforts, and provide opportunities and resources to those in need.

Essential Facts

Incidence and Prevalence

Incidence refers to the frequency of the disease or syndrome in a specific population.

Prevalence refers to the proportion of a specific population that has been impacted by the disease or syndrome at a distinct point in time.

Essential Facts

Factors That Influence Diagnostic Reliability, Validity and Classification Accuracy When Using the *Diagnostic and Statistical Manual of Mental Disorders*

- Data collection inconsistencies, time factor, and errors in self-administered questionaries and screenings
- Poor historian secondary to patient's state or ability to communicate
- Caretaker, guardian, or proxy's low health literacy, inability, or unwillingness
- Lack of clinician skill, experience, or training
- Atypical presentation of syndrome

Case Formulations

In psychiatry, case formulations or biopsychosocial formulations are a structured systematic approach toward methodologically conceptualizing and understanding the origin of a patient's symptom beyond a diagnostic label during a point in time. As the link between assessment and management, case formulations are descriptive integrations of the patient's information that help clinicians explore distinct, etiologic, behavioral, and treatment-prognostic dimensions and guide the course of treatment (Savander et al., 2019). Assessment based on case formulation enables clinicians to hypothesize about the origins, precipitants, and influences of a person's psychologic, interpersonal, and behavioral problems (Savander et al., 2019).

An astute clinician will systematically examine and decipher normal versus abnormal variations from presented assessment data to determine the severity of risk (prioritizing), identify problems, and denote symptoms of mental disorders captured by the *DSM-5* categories. This information helps clinicians formulate a diagnosis and initiate management (Savander et al., 2019). Unlike other medical specialties, definitive diagnostic tests and lab tests do not exist in psychiatry; therefore, a large part of the data is subjective or reported. Throughout the course of treatment, the data obtained from the interview, the physical assessment, and other diagnostic procedures are used to appraise diagnostic accuracy and course of treatment.

What Constitutes a Psychiatric Emergency?

The origin of what represents an emergency is danger. Suicide is a worldwide phenomenon impacting all populations; thus, suicide is the most common psychiatric emergency. Approximately 800,000 people die by suicide each year worldwide. Currently, data do not indicate that routine screenings for suicide reduce mortality (GBD 2015 Mortality and Causes of Death Collaborators, 2016; World Health Organization [WHO], 2021). Eighty percent of suicide victims had contact with a primary-care clinician within a year of their death (Stene-Larsen & Reneflot, 2019). Psychiatric emergencies can be difficult to identify; however, it is essential for all clinicians to screen and identify if a patient is demonstrating suicidal ideation, self-inflicted harm, or harm to others.

Warning signs of acute suicide risk include (a) threats, remarks, speaking, or writing about a desire or plan to hurt or kill oneself; (b) searching for a means to inflict harm or kill oneself (i.e., obtaining a gun or pills); and (c) engaging in unconventional activities that are out of the norm (American Association of Suicidology, n.d.). Clinicians must be prepared to recognize these warning signs to ensure safety to themselves, patients, and others. It is also important for clinicians to determine if a patient needs to be voluntarily or involuntarily detained for surveillance. Additional screening methods include reviewing a patient's past attempts, access to firearms, repeated thoughts of suicide or dying, self-harm behaviors, and substance abuse.

As cited in Potter et al. (2020), the Substance Abuse and Mental Health Services Administration (2009) developed the Five-Step Evaluation and Triage screening tool to identify suicide risk, severity, and protective factors. This tool assesses and documents (a) identifiable risk factors; (b) protective factors; (c) suicide inquiry, including thoughts, plans, and intent; (d) determination of risk or level of intervention; and (e) risk, plan, and follow-up (Table 1.4 Potter et al., 2020; Weber & Estes, 2016).

Psychiatric emergencies may include severe life-threatening events, such as abrupt behavioral changes that encompass (a) self-harm with or without suicidality; (b) homicide; (c) abuse; (d) severe psychomotor

Table 1.4

Suicide Screen: Mnemonic SAD PERSONS

SAD PERSONS Suicide Criteria	Scoring
S - Male	1 point
A - Age (<19 or >45 years)	1 point
D - Depression or hopelessness	2 points
P - Previous attempt or psychiatric care	1 point
E - Excessive alcohol or drug use	1 point
R - Rational thinking loss	2 points
S - Single, separated, divorced, or widowed	1 point
O - Organized previous suicide attempt	2 points
N - No social support	1 point
S - Stated future intent	2 points
Score 6–8 = emergency psychiatric evaluation; >9 immediate psychiatric hospitalization	

Source: Adapted from Patterson, W. M., Dohn, H. H., Bird, J., & Patterson, G. A. (1983). Evaluation of suicidal patients: The SAD PERSONS scale. *Psychosomatics, 24*, 343–345, 348–349. https://doi.org/10.1016/S0033-3182(83)73213-5

agitation; (e) catatonia; (f) anaphylaxis or allergic drug reactions; (g) toxic ingestion; (h) marked loss of consciousness; or (i) abrupt changes in cognition, delirium, psychosis, and abnormal vital signs (Wilson et al., 2017). Clinicians must determine if medical attention supplants psychiatric care in certain medical emergency situations.

Essential Facts

Key Points for Suicide Risk

- Perform ongoing risk assessment.
- Develop collaborative safety plan to manage suicidal behaviors.
- Establish care coordination protocols for rapid referrals to evidence-based suicide-specific care.
- Give attention to means reduction (firearms, substances, etc.).
- Enact consistent engagement efforts and cultivate connections.
- Offer continual support during high-risk periods.

(Stanley et al., 2018)

Essential Facts

There are two main categories of psychiatric emergency:

1. Acute psychomotor agitation
2. Suicidal or self-destructive behavior

Psychiatric emergencies require immediate intervention. The goal is to prevent harm or other serious consequences to patients and/or others. The main steps include (a) triage (environment, safety), (b) screening (underlying medical or neurologic cause of behavior), (c) assessment (intoxification, substance use or withdrawal, dementia), and (d) treatment (inpatient vs. outpatient).

It is of critical importance that contact with patients during an emergency prioritize safety for both the patient and the clinician.

Essential Facts

- Globally, suicides are the fourth leading cause of premature mortality in individuals aged 15 to 29 (WHO, 2021).
- Men complete suicide almost twice as often as women; however, women attempt suicide more often.
- Suicide rates were highest for men above 75 years old and lowest for those aged 10 to 14 (Centers for Disease Control and Prevention, 2020).
- Percentage of suicide attempts is 10 to 30 times higher than completed suicides (Bachmann, 2018).
- Mental health illness increases the risk for completed suicides by 98% (Bachmann, 2018).
- Mood disorders account for one-third of fatal suicide attempts.
- The most predictive factors for suicide are associated with suicide ideation, non-suicidal self-injurious behaviors and prior suicide attempts (Fosse et al., 2017).

Essential Facts

Codeterminants and Protective Factors

Codeterminants of increased suicide risk:

- Demographics
- Social status
- Social change
- Community
- Environment

(*continued*)

Essential Facts (*continued*)

- Chronic physical and mental illnesses
- Abuse of alcohol and substances
- Previous attempts

Protective factors:

- Absence of risk factors
- Past history of self-control
- Cultural or religious beliefs that are against suicide
- Fears of letting down others
- Safety planning

(Stanley et al., 2018; Welton, 2007).

Essential Facts

Suicide Assessment Mnemonic

IS PATH WARM?

- (Suicide) ideation (SI): Reports SI, or desire to kill oneself? Purchase or access to a gun or other weapon?
- Substance abuse: Heightened or new onset of alcohol or drug usage?
- Purposelessness: Expresses a lack or loss of purpose or a reason to live?
- Anger: Does the client express feelings of rage or uncontrolled anger? Expresses wanting revenge against others? Intense anger or rage, blaming of others?
- Trapped: Feelings of being trapped or stuck? Feelings of agony or pain? Feeling that death is the only solution?
- Hopelessness: A negative sense of self, others, and future? Expresses hopelessness?
- Withdrawing: Indicates the desire to withdraw from family, friends, and society? Isolates self?
- Anxiety: Feelings of anxiousness, agitation, or unable to sleep? Lacks ability to relax? Increased sleep or poor sleep quality?
- Recklessness: Reckless or engages in risky activities, seemingly without considering consequences?
- Mood change: Reported dramatic mood shifts or states?

(American Association of Suicidology, n.d.)

SUMMARY

Structured interviews, semistructured interviews, and questionnaires have become the gold standard for diagnostic interviewing for psychiatric mental health assessments across populations. Psychiatric evaluations are a diagnostic tool employed by mental health clinicians to collect patient information and assess for anomalies of experience, belief, thought process, expression, behavior, and overall functioning. This information is useful in helping clinicians determine if symptoms are present, assess the severity of the symptoms, formulate a diagnosis, triage patient needs, plan an appropriate course of treatment, and guide ongoing clinical decisions. It is essential that clinicians assess severe symptoms requiring immediate intervention, such as suicidal behaviors, harmful gestures to self or others, delusions, hallucinations, or acute disturbance in thought, behavior, and/or mood. It is also important to consider the patient's mental and physical health throughout psychiatric examinations.

REVIEW QUESTIONS

1. What the drug does to the body is referred to as which one of the following?
   a. Pharmacologic distribution
   b. Pharmacokinetics
   c. Pharmacodynamics
   d. Pharmacoregulation
2. Which one of the following statements is true?
   a. Men attempt suicide more than females and have fewer suicide-related deaths.
   b. The percentage of suicide attempts is 10 to 30 times higher than completed suicides.
   c. Predictive factors for suicide include being a White male with no prior attempts.
   d. Suicide assessments are only performed during the initial interview.
3. *Reliability* refers to which one of the following?
   a. Consistency of a measure and the ability to reproduce results under equivalent conditions
   b. The extent to which the results really measure what they are intended to measure
   c. An operational systematic process for defining variable indicators
   d. Tests wherein the purpose is clear
4. During the termination stage of the therapeutic relationship, which one of the following occurs?
   a. Key principles are effective communication, trust, and honesty.
   b. The therapist suggests self-management strategies.
   c. The therapist and patient establish goals.
   d. Issues and challenges are identified and problem-solving skills are developed.
5. Which one of the following statements is accurate?
   a. *Sensitivity* refers to those who have a disease test negative, and *specificity* refers to those who do have the disease test negative.
   b. *Sensitivity* refers to the false-positive rate, and *specificity* refers to those who do not have the disease test positive.
   c. *Sensitivity* refers to those who have a disease test positive or true positive rate, and *specificity* refers to those who do not have the disease, test negative, or the true negative rate.
   d. The *DSM-5* has a high sensitivity and specificity.

REFERENCES

Aboraya, A., Nasrallah, H., Muvvala, S., El-Missiry, A., Mansour, H., Hill, C., Elswick, D., & Price, E. C. (2016). The Standard for Clinicians' Interview in Psychiatry (SCIP): A clinician-administered tool with categorical, dimensional, and numeric output—Conceptual development, design, and description of the SCIP. *Innovations in Clinical Neuroscience, 13*(5–6), 31–77. https://www.ncbi.nlm.nih.gov/pmc/articles/PMC5077257

Allen, M. L., Cook, B. L., Carson, N., Interian, A., La Roche, M., & Alegría, M. (2017). Patient-provider therapeutic alliance contributes to patient activation in community mental health clinics. *Administration and Policy in Mental Health, 44*(4), 431–440. https://doi.org/10.1007/s10488-015-0655-8

American Psychiatric Association. (2013). *Diagnostic and statistical manual of mental disorders* (5th ed.). https://doi.org/10.1176/appi.books.9780890425596

American Psychiatric Association. (2016). *The American Psychiatric Association practice guidelines for the psychiatric evaluation of adults* (3rd ed.). American Psychiatric Association.

Bachmann, S. (2018). Epidemiology of suicide and the psychiatric perspective. *International Journal of Environmental Research and Public Health, 15*(7), Article 1425. https://doi.org/10.3390/ijerph15071425

Centers for Disease Control and Prevention. (2020). *Increase in suicide mortality in the United States, 1999–2018* (Data Brief No. 362). https://www.cdc.gov/nchs/products/databriefs/db362.htm

Fosse, R., Ryberg, W., Carlsson, M. K., & Hammer, J. (2017, March 16). Predictors of suicide in the patient population admitted to a locked-door psychiatric acute ward. *PLOS ONE, 12*(3), e0173958. https://doi.org/10.1371/journal.pone.0173958

GBD 2015 Mortality and Causes of Death Collaborators. (2016). Global, regional, and national life expectancy, all-cause mortality, and cause-specific mortality for 249 causes of death, 1980–2015: A systematic analysis for the global burden of disease study 2015. *Lancet, 388*(10053), 1459–1544. https://doi.org/10.1016/S0140-6736(16)31012-1

Johnson, K., & Vanderhoef, D. (2016). *Review and resource manual: Psychiatric mental health nurse practitioner.* American Nurses Association.

McLeod, B. D., Jensen-Doss, A., Tully, C. B., Southam-Gerow, M. A., Weisz, J. R., & Kendall, P. C. (2016). The role of setting versus treatment type in alliance within youth therapy. *Journal of Consulting and Clinical Psychology, 84*(5), 453–464. https://doi.org/10.1037/ccp0000081

Nordgaard, J., Sass, L. A., & Parnas, J. (2013). The psychiatric interview: Validity, structure, and subjectivity. *European Archives of Psychiatry and Clinical Neuroscience, 263*(4), 353–364. https://doi.org/10.1007/s00406-012-0366-z

Potter, D. R., Stockdale, S., & O'Mallon, M. (2020). A case study approach: Psychopharmacology for atypical antidepressants snap shot. *International Journal of Caring Sciences, 13*(1), 764–769. https://www.internationaljournalofcaringsciences.org/docs/85_potter_original_13_1.pdf

Savander, E., Weiste, E., Hintikka, J., Leiman, M., Valkeapää, T., Heinonen, E., & Peräkylä, A. (2019). Offering patients opportunities to reveal their subjective experiences in psychiatric assessment interviews. *Patient Education and Counseling, 102*(7), 1296–1303. https://doi.org//10.1016/j.pec.2019.02.021

Stanley, B., Brown, G. K., Brenner, L. A., Galfalvy, H. C., Currier, G. W., Knox, K. L., Chaudhury, S. R., Bush, A. L., & Green, K. L. (2018). Comparison of the safety planning intervention with follow-up vs usual care of suicidal patients treated in the emergency department. *JAMA Psychiatry, 75*(9), 894–900. https://doi.org/10.1001/jamapsychiatry.2018.1776

Stene-Larsen, K., & Reneflot, A. (2019). Contact with primary and mental health care prior to suicide: A systematic review of the literature from 2000 to 2017. *Scandinavian Journal of Public Health, 47*(1), 9–17. https://doi.org/10.1177/1403494817746274

Stiles, J., & Jernigan, T. L. (2010). The basics of brain development. *Neuropsychology Review, 20*(4), 327–348. https://doi.org/10.1007/s11065-010-9148-4

Substance Abuse and Mental Health Services Administration (SAMHSA.) (2009)

Weber, M., & Estes, K. (2016). Anxiety and depression. In T. Woo & M. V. Robinson (Eds.), *Pharmacotherapeutics: For advanced practice nurse prescribers* (pp. 897–912). F. A. Davis.

Welton, R. S. (2007). The management of suicidality: Assessment and intervention. *Psychiatry (Edgmont), 4*(5), 24–34. https://www.ncbi.nlm.nih.gov/pmc/articles/PMC2921310

World Health Organization. (2021). *Suicide.* https://www.who.int/news-room/fact-sheets/detail/suicide

Wilson, M. P., Nordstrom, K., Anderson, E. L., Ng, A. T., Zun, L. S., Peltzer-Jones, J. M., & Allen, M. H. (2017). American Association for Emergency Psychiatry task force on medical clearance of adult psychiatric patients. Part II: Controversies over medical assessment, and consensus recommendations. *Western Journal of Emergency Medicine, 18*(4), 640–646. https://doi.org/10.5811/westjem.2017.3.32259

2

The Prescriber's Role

Communication impacts all levels of care, including diagnostic accuracy, treatment, monitoring, and clinical outcomes. Clinicians use bidirectional communication and interpersonal skills to obtain information, facilitate care, provide counsel, and establish therapeutic relationships. Patient–provider communication and interactions contribute to increased patient adherence and positive health outcomes. The clinician's verbal and nonverbal communication is important during the psychiatric interview and can impact pertinent information sharing, delivery of diagnosis, and other therapeutic processes (McCabe & Healey, 2018).

In this chapter you will learn:

1. The importance of communication during psychiatric interviews
2. How to use nonverbal and verbal communication to establish rapport
3. The components of patient-centered care
4. How to identify cultural implications for care
5. The domains of informed consent
6. How to use evidence-based medication management considerations

COMMUNICATION

Diagnostic accuracy in psychiatry is dependent on patients' observable signs and reported symptoms; therefore, clinician interview and communication skills are key to psychiatry. The dyadic relationship between the clinician and the patient is established when interviews are conducted with warm and welcoming approaches. Clinicians must foster trust early for essential information exchanges to occur. Early during the interview, clinicians should inquire about the patient's chief complaint and allow the patient to share their thoughts. This inquiry enables the clinician to assess body language, speech, posturing, facial expressions, thoughts, and insight. Open-ended questions or statements prompt the patient to speak freely so thought coherence and connectedness can be assessed. Moreover, attentive listening, genuine curiosity, validation, and empathic questioning can enable feelings of being "heard" that can help the clinician acquire a deeper understanding of the patient's needs and expectations. In addition, offering reflective statements or summaries can encourage patients to briefly tell their stories. Clinicians should assess patients' areas of support and stressors, including functional impairments as well as work, academic, financial, and social interactions.

Clinicians can use open-ended and closed-ended follow-up questioning to clarify or expand thoughts and ideas that can be used to guide diagnosis and management. Effective communication and self-awareness are interconnected; therefore, it is important for clinicians to continuously consider their actions and how they are being perceived throughout the interview. To improve your relationship-building skills and establish the patient's trust, use the acronyms PEARLS and EMPOWERS (see Table 2.1; Barnett, 2001; Dickert & Kass, 2009).

Patient-centered communication is an approach that emphasizes shared decision-making or partnering with the patient and caregiver. Clinicians using patient-centered communication create a personalized treatment approach that aligns with the patient's concerns, preferences, physical and cognitive capacities, and the biologic, psychologic, and social features of the illness that are unique to the individual (McCabe & Healey, 2018). Patient-centered dialogue is a core component of psychiatric interviews and intended to gather information to provide applicable care, understand the patient's perception of their illness, and gain the patient's trust. Table 2.2 lists the principles of patient-centered care.

Table 2.1

Relationship-Building Mnemonics

PEARLS	EMPOWERS
Partnership: develop a treatment plan together	**E**mpathy: show understanding of feelings
Empathy: show understanding of experience	**M**anage session time and goals
Apology/acknowledgment: show concern	**P**erspective of patient sharing of ideas
Respect: pay attention to specific needs and recognize individuality and autonomy	**O**bservation summary of patient
Legitimization: reassure or validate their feelings	**W**ork on a plan as partners
Support: remind patients that you are there to help them	**E**mpower goals and dedication to plan
	Reach for client/patient decision-making
	Summarize concerns and observations

Source: Adapted from Dickert, N. W., & Kass, N. E. (2009). Understanding respect: Learning from patients. *Journal of Medical Ethics*, *35*(7), 419–423. https://doi.org/10.1136/jme.2008.027235. Copyright 2009 by British Medical Association; Barnett, P. B. (2001). Rapport and the hospitalist. *American Journal of Medicine*, *111*(9 Suppl. 2), 31S–35S. https://doi.org/10.1016/s0002-9343(01)00967-6

Table 2.2

Principles of Patient-Centered Care
1. Access
2. Respect for patient's preferences
3. Coordination of care and services
4. Physical comfort and well-being
5. Emotional support
6. Inclusion of family, caregivers, and other support
7. Education and information access
8. Transition and continuity

Essential Facts

For children and older adults with cognitive impairments, reports often rely upon parents and caregivers; therefore, considerations for altered perceptions should be considered.

Rating scales completed by patients, parents, caregivers, and teachers can be used to determine severity of symptoms and to assess for inconsistencies in reporting.

Clinicians can use follow-up questioning to clarify unclear or vague comments. Follow-up statements or questions can also be used to promote accountability or demonstrate levels of commitment to treatment. Supportive and empathic questioning that asks for clarification or expands on specific topic areas is used to avoid inaccurate, diminished, or exaggerated reporting. It is important that clinicians assess for inaccurate reporting due to concerns such as stigma, fear, misinterpretation of normal versus abnormal behaviors, and lack of insight. Clinicians should also acquire consent to obtain collateral reports or to review previous medical records to promote diagnostic accuracy.

Essential Facts

Strategies for Follow-Up Questioning

- Empathy is the ability to recognize and fathom the patient's situation, including their perspective, beliefs, and experiences.
- Nonverbal communication or nonlinguistic communication exchanges may include facial expressions, eye contact, posture, positioning of oneself, and touch.
- Microexpressions are brief involuntary facial expressions that occur when experiencing an emotion, such as eyebrow or lip corner movements.

The main objectives for the psychiatric interview include (a) establishing rapport or trust and (b) making inquiries about chief complaint(s) and history of the present illness to explore the interconnection between biologic, psychologic, and socioenvironmental factors that influence a patient's symptoms. As feelings, thoughts, past and present stressors, and other problems are expressed, the clinician identifies and measures the severity and patterns of symptoms to understand the patient's underlying psychopathology and make evidence-based clinical decisions. Patient safety assessments are ongoing throughout the interview.

Clinicians can use rating scales or validated clinical measurement instruments to objectively assess, treat, and manage clinical outcomes, including efficacy of treatment, safety, tolerability, functioning, and quality of life in patients (Aboraya et al., 2016). Toward the end of the psychiatric interview, clinicians should provide feedback, recognize patients' strengths, initiate the treatment plan, reframe misconceptions, mitigate concerns, and provide detailed follow-up and safety information and resources. During the psychiatry assessment, the clinician should (a) identify the interconnections between the biologic, psychologic, and socioenvironmental factors that influence the patient's symptoms and (b) assess for safety and comorbidities.

MOTIVATION FOR TREATMENT

Common factors for treatment motivation include the therapeutic alliance, adherence or compliance of recommendations, and an intrinsic drive or motivation for behavior change. Personal motivating factors result from positive personal experiences of culture, intrinsic values, and genuine interest in health-related outcomes. Motivation is a key mechanism toward change because increased levels of motivation lead to treatment entry, increased retention rates, improved self-care behaviors, and improved psychologic and overall functioning for patients with psychiatric disorders.

CULTURAL IMPLICATIONS FOR TREATMENT

To foster therapeutic relationships, clinicians should consider sociocultural differences, such as language barriers and differences in health-related beliefs, that may lead to mistrust, dissatisfaction, decreased adherence, and poorer health outcomes. The consideration of cultural, linguistic, religious, sexual, and racial or ethnic characteristics of patients, caregivers, and team members is integral to proficient and culturally sensitive communication. Furthermore, clinicians who assess the individual cultural factors that influence patients' perceptions of their symptoms and treatment options can build an all-inclusive foundation to accurately diagnose and deliver a patient-centered and culturally sensitive treatment plan (American Psychiatric Association, 2013).

Essential Facts

About Culture-Bound Syndromes

- They are distinct behavioral, affective, and cognitive manifestations linked to a person's culture and not to a psychiatric disorder.
- Due to increasing globalization, "culture bound" syndromes are being seen by clinicians in different cultures and geographical regions.
- Cultural assessments provide an understanding of the client's narrative since subjective experiences depend on personal, social, and cultural context.

HEALTH LITERACY

Mental health clinicians have a responsibility to provide patient information that is accessible and understandable. In addition, patients with increased health literacy show increased levels of treatment-seeking and adherence to recommended interventions; thus, health literacy is one of the pivotal determinants in population health outcomes. Health literacy refers to the cognitive and social skills that patients need to understand, appraise, and apply health information to make informed and safe decisions about their health (Rolova et al., 2020; Sørensen et al., 2012). Clinicians can increase patients' health literacy by speaking with plain language, using standardized health communication tools, engaging in face-to-face communication and drawings, and involving staff, interpreters, and caregivers in discussions.

INFORMED CONSENT

Providing information to patients about their medication is a fundamental responsibility of clinicians. Medication information is expected to be provided in written, verbal, or both forms. Informed consent is a requisite for the protection of patient rights and interests, and this practice is rooted in the ethical principles of respect and autonomy. Informed consent refers to the voluntary acceptance of medical care by a cognitively competent patient after the disclosure of the plan, likely consequences, risks, benefits, and alternative treatment options. Informed consent is an active process that engages patients—both adults and children—in healthcare decisions. In informed consent, clinicians must disclose information to cognitively competent patients and their surrogates to obtain legal authorization before undertaking any health-related interventions (Amer, 2013). It is important for clinicians to acknowledge that, over time, children and adolescents may develop their own opinions about their own medical decision-making due to developmental maturation. In addition, clinicians can incorporate cost considerations and culturally sensitive management to better incorporate family values in the informed consent (Amer, 2013; Katz et al., 2016). Table 2.3 lists

Table 2.3

Five Key Elements of Informed Consent

Voluntarism	Acts voluntarily without being subjected to the control and influence of others
Competency	Has capacity to understand and to act reasonably in their judgment
Disclosure	A professional practice standard—disclosure of information typically provided A reasonable person standard—disclosure of information relevant to a decision A subjective standard—disclosure of information that must be made by a specific person
Understanding	Has ability to comprehend the information given
Decision	Patient's or surrogates' voluntary authorization

Table 2.4

Exceptions to Informed Consent Requirement in Adult Psychiatry

Necessity	A circumstance in which grave harm or death is likely to occur without intervention and there is some uncertainty about the patient's competence
Emergency situations	A circumstance when the patient is incapable of providing consent and a surrogate is not available to provide the consent, yet there is a danger to the patient's life or danger of serious health impairment and immediate intervention is necessary to avert this danger.

the five key elements of informed consent, and Table 2.4 lists the exceptions to informed consent requirements in adult psychiatry.

GUIDING PRINCIPLES IN PSYCHOPHARMACOLOGY AND MEDICATION MANAGEMENT ROLE

Pharmacologic refers to the use of psychotropic medication to treat psychiatric disorders. The balance between treating mental health symptoms and avoiding medication-related harm is a critical objective for mental health professionals and can be challenging to achieve in clinical practice. Once a diagnosis is derived and target symptoms are identified, clinicians must consider the stage of the illness (acute, relapse, chronic), comorbidities, economic status, coexisting medical conditions, compliance issues, side effect profile, previous treatment response, timely follow-up, adjusting medications according to treatment response, and appearing side effects. It is essential that clinicians partner with the patient and tailor prescribed medications to meet the patient's individual needs and achieve optimal compliance and better health outcomes. Clinicians should also consider the known tolerability and safety profiles of psychotropic medications that may be prescribed separately or in conjunction with psychotherapy or other services to eliminate or alleviate symptoms of psychiatric disorders. Whenever possible, psychotropic medications should be prescribed second line (when psychotherapy or other services produce an inadequate response) or in conjunction with evidence-based psychotherapies or support services. Clinicians must be mindful of patients' personal values, needs, and preferences and explore hesitation and misconceptions of information. Clinicians should use plain language, provide patients with education about their illness, discuss the potential benefits and risks of medication, and explain the alternative options that are available. The patient's decision-making should also be informed by details about the known serious side effects associated with medication use. Duration is an important dosing instruction, especially with psychotropic medications; therefore, clinicians must consider the illness and emphasize the need to continue medication for the long term when applicable.

Essential Facts

General Patient-Specific Psychotropic Prescribing Considerations

- Associated morbidities (medical/surgical/psychiatric/substance use, etc.)
- Gender (male/female)
- Lab values (liver functions, renal functions, medical conditions, other unique attributes, etc.)
- Medication allergies
- Patient's age (geriatric/middle aged/pediatric)
- Probable side effects of drugs
- Weight

Essential Facts

General Psychotropic Management Considerations

- Adjust medication as indicated based on symptom reduction and treatment goals.
- Avoid medications that may result in dependency and educate patients about associated risks.
- Avoid polypharmacy.
- Assess environmental factors and safety.
- Assess for pregnancy and pregnancy planning (in some circumstances, risk vs. benefit may be indicated as well as collaboration with obstetrician).

(continued)

Essential Facts (*continued*)

- Assess the patient's knowledge of previously prescribed and/or over-the-counter medication(s) including name(s), dose(s), route(s), schedule(s) and purpose(s).
- Consult with family, caregiver, pharmacist, and/or other health care professionals to confirm medication list accuracy.
- Communicate dosing instructions (name, strength, frequency, duration, route of administration).
- Document informed consent and understanding.
- Review U.S. Food and Drug Administration (FDA) indication for medication.
- Identify possible interactions of prescribed medications.
- Inform patients about possible signs and symptoms of adverse side effects and possible undesirable effects.
- Monitor medication response.
- Monitor effectiveness of prescribed medications on symptoms reduction.
- Monitor side effects (scales may be helpful).
- Mutually determine length of care.
- Obtain family history and previous medication responses of family members.
- Prioritize reduction of adverse effects.
- Provide reliable and attainable resources.
- Set a schedule of drugs.
- Strive to prescribe the least amount of medication at the lowest effective dose.
- (Re)organize medication list to secure medication accuracy.

Essential Facts

- Polypharmacy, the use of five or more medications by an individual, is more commonly found in adults older than the age of 65; however, clinicians need to consider its risks in all patients.
- Recent data indicate that approximately 39% of older adults in the United States take five or more medications (Rankin et al., 2018).

SUMMARY

Patient-centered care considers an individual's values, beliefs, and spiritual and cultural practices. Therapeutic communication and interpersonal skills are essential to gaining patients' trust, facilitating care, establishing therapeutic relationships, safeguarding diagnostic accuracy and treatment, monitoring conditions, and counseling to promote resilience to help patients manage the after-effects of distressing circumstances. Providing accessible and understandable information to patients and/or caregivers about diagnosis, medication, and/or treatment planning is a fundamental responsibility of mental health clinicians.

REVIEW QUESTIONS

1. Exceptions to informed consent requirements in adult psychiatry include which one of the following?
   a. A circumstance in which serious harm or death is likely to occur without the intervention, and during an emergency circumstance when the patient is incapable of providing consent and a surrogate is not available to provide the consent.
   b. A circumstance in which grave harm or death is not likely to occur without the intervention, and during an emergency circumstance when the patient is capable of providing consent and a surrogate is available to provide the consent.
   c. There is danger to the patient's life or danger of serious health impairment and immediate intervention is necessary to avert this danger and harm or death is not likely to occur without the intervention.
   d. None of the above are correct.
2. Which one of the following is not included in the informed consent?
   a. Voluntarism
   b. Negotiation
   c. Competency
   d. Understanding
3. Which one of the following statements is correct?
   a. Whenever possible, psychotropic medications should be prescribed first line, before psychotherapy.
   b. Personal values, needs, and preferences should not be considered in prescribing psychotropic medications.
   c. Whenever possible, use medical jargon to provide education about their illness, as well as potential benefits and risks of medication.
   d. Use plain language to provide education about their illness, potential benefits and risks of medication, and alternative options, if available.
4. Informed consents are rooted in which one of the following ethical principles?
   a. Respect and autonomy
   b. Respect and promises
   c. Guarantees and respect
   d. Autonomy and loyalty
5. Once a diagnosis has been made and target symptoms are identified, the prescriber needs to consider which one of the following?
   a. The stage of the illness (acute, relapse, chronic)
   b. Comorbidities, economic status, and coexisting medical conditions
   c. Compliance issues, side-effect profile, and previous treatment response
   d. All of the above are correct.

REFERENCES

Aboraya, A., Nasrallah, H., Muvvala, S., El-Missiry, A., Mansour, H., Hill, C., Elswick, D., & Price, E. C. (2016). The Standard for Clinicians' Interview in Psychiatry (SCIP): A clinician-administered tool with categorical, dimensional, and numeric output—conceptual development, design, and description of the SCIP. *Innovations in Clinical Neuroscience*, *13*(5–6), 31–77. https://www.ncbi.nlm.nih.gov/pmc/articles/PMC5077257

Amer, A. B. (2013). Informed consent in adult psychiatry. *Oman Medical Journal*, *28*(4), 228–231. https://doi.org/10.5001/omj.2013.67

American Psychiatric Association. (2013). *Diagnostic and statistical manual of mental disorders* (5th ed.). https://doi.org/10.1176/appi.books.9780890425596

Barnett, P. B. (2001). Rapport and the hospitalist. *American Journal of Medicine*, *111*(9 Suppl. 2), 31S–35S. https://doi.org/10.1016/s0002-9343(01)00967-6

Dickert, N. W., & Kass, N. E. (2009). Understanding respect: Learning from patients. *Journal of Medical Ethics*, *35*(7), 419–423. https://doi.org/10.1136/jme.2008.027235

Katz, A. L., Webb, S. A., & Committee on Bioethics. (2016). Informed consent in decision-making in pediatric practice. *Pediatrics*, *138*(2), Article e20161485. https://doi.org/10.1542/peds.2016-1485

McCabe, R., & Healey, P. (2018). Miscommunication in doctor-patient communication. *Topics in Cognitive Science*, *10*(2), 409–424. https://doi.org/10.1111/tops.12337

Rankin, A., Cadogan, C. A., Patterson, S. M., Kerse, N., Cardwell, C. R., Bradley, M. C., Ryan, C., & Hughes, C. (2018). Interventions to improve the appropriate use of polypharmacy for older people. *Cochrane Database of Systematic Reviews*, *9*(9), Article CD008165. https://doi.org/10.1002/14651858.CD008165.pub4

Rolova, G., Gavurova, B., & Petruzelka, B. (2020). Exploring health literacy in individuals with alcohol addiction: A mixed methods clinical study. *International Journal of Environmental Research and Public Health*, *17*(18), Article 6728. https://doi.org/10.3390/ijerph17186728

Sørensen, K., Van den Broucke, S., Fullam, J., Doyle, G., Pelikan, J., Slonska, Z., Brand, H., & (HLS-EU) Consortium Health Literacy Project European. (2012). Health literacy and public health: A systematic review and integration of definitions and models. *BMC Public Health*, 12, Article 80. https://doi.org/10.1186/1471-2458-12-80

3

The Brain and Nervous System

The brain is a massive network that contains billions of cells and nerve fibers. Due to the brain's interconnectedness to vital organ systems and its complicated neuroanatomy, it is considered to be the most complex organ within the body. For decades, scientists have tried to comprehend how the brain and nervous system function. In fact, neurochemical transmission was recognized prior to the 1950s, and scientists believed that central nervous system neurons communicated through electrical impulses (Braslow & Marder, 2019). This chapter highlights the brain's major structures and provides an overview of the central and peripheral nervous systems, basic concepts of neurotransmission, and general principles of pharmacology.

In this chapter you will learn:

1. To identify the structures of the major brain regions
2. To comprehend the sensory and motor system connections to the brain
3. To develop an understanding of the basic structure and function of the nervous system
4. To identify basic neural cellular structures
5. To conceptualize common principles in psychopharmacology

MAIN STRUCTURES OF THE BRAIN

The structural anatomy of the brain is complex; however, it can be broken down into simple concepts that are easy to understand. For simplicity, we will divide the brain into three basic anatomical parts: the brainstem, the cerebellum, and the cerebrum (left and right cerebral hemispheres).

Table 3.1

Brainstem Key Terms: Structure

Brain Structure	Function
Pons	Consists of nuclei that relay signals from the forebrain to the cerebellum that regulate sleep, respiration, swallowing, bladder control, hearing, equilibrium, taste, eye movement, facial expressions, facial sensation, and posture
Medulla oblongata (myelencephalon)	Regulates autonomic, involuntary functions (breathing, heart rate, and blood pressure) through vasomotor centers
Midbrain (mesencephalon)	Impacts motor control, sleep and wake cycles, alertness, vision and hearing, temperature regulation

THE BRAINSTEM

The brainstem is a conduit for many ascending and descending pathways that are essential for many integrative functions, along with the body's vital functions. The brainstem is the structure that controls people's innate and automatic self-preserving behavior patterns; therefore, the brainstem is referred to as the "primal brain," "reptilian brain," or "trunk" of the brain. The brainstem consists of three parts: (a) the pons, (b) the medulla oblongata, and (c) the midbrain (see Table 3.1). At the brainstem, nerve connections from the motor and sensory systems of the cortex communicate with the peripheral nervous system. The brainstem is the structure responsible for the regulation of cardiac (blood pressure) and respiratory function (breathing), digestion, control of movement, consciousness, impulse control, cognition, modulation of pain, autonomic reflexes, arousal, memory, and sleep cycle.

Essential Facts

Ridges and grooves located in the brain serve to increase the brain's surface area and are referred to as *fissures* and *sulci*.

- *Sulci* are the small grooves or depressions in the cerebral cortex. The larger grooves are called *fissures*.
- The *gyri* are the ridges or bulges between the grooves and are responsible for the brain's wrinkled appearance.

CEREBELLUM

The cerebellum, sometimes referred to as the "little brain," obtains information from the balance system of the inner ear, sensory nerves, and the auditory and visual systems. The cerebellum is traditionally considered to be part of the motor system and is responsible for control and coordination of voluntary movement. Additionally, evidence indicates that functions of the cerebellum include task domains, such as memory, language, emotion, and perceptual functions; however, its role beyond motor control is not well understood (Baumann et al., 2015). Motor commands are not initiated in the cerebellum; rather, through signal processing, the cerebellum modifies motor commands from descending pathways to make movements accurate and more adaptive. Notably, damage to the cerebellum leads to impairments in motor control and posture.

Essential Facts

Cerebellum Functions

- Balance and equilibrium
- Cognition
- Control and coordination of movement
- Emotion and perceptual functions
- Fine motor coordination
- Impulse control
- Language
- Memory
- Motor learning
- Posture

CEREBRUM

The cerebrum, also referred to as the forebrain, is the largest structure of the brain. The cerebrum contains two cerebral hemispheres: the right hemisphere and the left hemisphere. Each hemisphere can be further divided into four lobes: (a) frontal, (b) temporal, (c) parietal, and (d) occipital. Each lobe comprises billions of neurons, glia, grey matter, and white matter.

Essential Facts

- The *grey matter* gets its color from a high concentration of neuronal cell bodies that contain the genes of the cell and are responsible for metabolism and synthesizing proteins. The expression "use your grey matter" is used to get a person to think harder.
- The *white matter* gets its color from myelin (a fatty white substance), which coats the axons of the neurons to protect them.
- Loss of either *grey or white matter* result in deficits in language, memory, reasoning, and other mental functions; both are vital to optimal brain functioning.

The great longitudinal fissure separates the two hemispheres; however, the hemispheres are connected at the *corpus callosum*. This connection creates routes or pathways for messaging between the hemispheres. Distinct fissures act as landmarks to divide the two hemispheres into the four lobes. Although the lobes are interconnected, each lobe has a distinct function (see Table 3.2). The cerebrum also includes the limbic system, often referred to as the emotional brain because it is the part of the brain that involves behavioral and emotional responses (see Table 3.3).

Table 3.2

Four Main Lobes of the Brain's Cerebral Cortex

Brain Structure	Function
Temporal lobe	Processes auditory input into emotional context; responsible for comprehending meaningful sounds and language; memory
Parietal lobe	Processes sensory information; integrates touch, taste, pain, pressure, temperature, spatial awareness, language processing
Occipital lobe	Visual processing of information; responsible for comprehending visual information; receives and interprets information from the eye's retinas
Frontal lobe	The emotional control center; personality; decision-making, planning, organization, and executive functioning; mood expression; attention; reward; short-term memory; motivation; and planning; houses the majority of dopamine-sensitive neurons

Table 3.3

Overview of the Limbic System Structure and Functions

Brain Structure	Function
Amygdala	Key role in emotional processing; fear, stress response ("fight or flight" response), emotional-affective dimension of pain and pain modulation, emotional memory, anxiety, worry, aggression, placidity, fear conditioning, rage
Hippocampus	Memory; formation, organization, and storage of new memories; connecting certain feelings and emotions to older memories; spatial memories
Thalamus	Relays (gatekeeper or relay station) sensory (except smell) and motor signals, as well as regulates of consciousness and alertness; sleep and wakefulness; processing and interpretation as touch, pain, or temperature; plays a vital role in projecting information from the basal ganglia to the motor cortex and back
Hypothalamus	Regulates the autonomic nervous system via hormone production and release; secondarily regulates blood pressure, heart rate, hunger, thirst, and sexual arousal; regulates the circadian sleep/wake cycle

BASAL GANGLIA

The *basal ganglia,* or the *corpus striatum* (striped body), refers to a group of subcortical nuclei primarily responsible for motor control, executive functions, behaviors, and emotions. This structure includes the *caudate*, *putamen*, and *globus pallidus*, all of which play a role in involuntary motor activities, such as muscle tone, posture, and reflexes. For example, syndromes that involve the basal ganglia include dementia, Huntington's disease, and Parkinson's disease.

Essential Facts

- The *left hemisphere* controls the *contralateral* (opposite) right side of the body, and is referred to as the "logical side" of the brain (analytical functioning, thought, reasoning).
- The *right hemisphere* controls the *contralateral* (opposite) left side of the body and is often referred to as the "creative side" of the brain (creativity, imagination, insight).
- Due to the basal ganglia's *extrapyramidal* motor nerve tracts and systems, psychotropic medications can impact the area, resulting in involuntary movement side effects.
- Extrapyramidal motor disease is generally characterized by impaired motor control, which is usually the result of basal ganglionic dysfunction.

CONCEPTS OF THE NERVOUS SYSTEM

The *central nervous system* (CNS), referred to as the body's control system, consists of the brain, spinal cord, grey matter, and white matter. The CNS controls breathing, heart rate, the release of hormones, body temperature, thoughts, movements, and emotions. The *peripheral nervous system* (PNS) contains all the nerves that lie outside of the CNS. The PNS connects the CNS to the body's organs, limbs, and skin so information can be transferred from the brain and spinal cord to and from other areas of the body. The PNS is divided into the *somatic nervous system* and *the autonomic nervous system* (see Table 3.4). Table 3.5 details cranial nerves and their functions.

BASIC NEUROPHYSIOLOGY

The human nervous system is a highly complex structure composed of many different cell structures that are essential for proper functioning. The major function of the nervous system is to transfer and exchange information. *Neurotransmission* is the process of transferring information from one nerve cell (neuron) to another. Neurons need to communicate with one another to transmit signals throughout the body. Each nerve cell contains a cell body (*soma*) that includes the *nucleus* and *axon* (stem or larger branching fiber)

Table 3.4

Somatic Nervous System and Autonomic Nervous Systems

Somatic Nervous System	Autonomic Nervous System
Carries sensory and motor information to and from the CNS (motor and sensory neurons)	Regulates involuntary body functions (parasympathetic system and sympathetic system)
Transmits sensory information	Blood flow
Assists voluntary movement	Heartbeat
	Digestion
	Breathing
	Fight-or-flight response

CNS, central nervous system.

Table 3.5

Cranial Nerves and Functions

Cranial Nerves and Functions	Sensory and/or Motor
Olfactory: Smell	Sensory
Optic: Visual fields and vision	Sensory
Oculomotor: Eye movements; eyelid opening	Motor
Trochlear: Eye movements (down and inward)	Motor
Trigeminal: Facial sensation; mastication muscles	Sensory and Motor
Abducens: Eye movements (lateral)	Motor
Facial: Eyelid and mouth closing; saliva and tears; facial expression; taste	Sensory and Motor
Auditory/vestibular: Hearing; balance	Sensory
Glossopharyngeal: Taste; swallow control	Sensory and Motor
Vagus: Swallowing; taste; carotid reflex	Sensory and Motor
Accessory: Neck and shoulder muscle control	Motor
Hypoglossal: Movement of tongue	Motor

covered by *myelin sheath* and *dendrites* (smaller branching fibers) that collect incoming signals to send to the neuron's cell body. *Synapses* refer to intercellular junctions that connect the presynaptic terminals of axons with the postsynaptic dendrites of other neurons (Shin et al., 2019).

Neurotransmitters are stored in synaptic vesicles prior to being released. *Action potentials* within the axon release neurotransmitters into the *synaptic cleft,* an opening at the end of each neuron that enables electrical or chemical signals to pass over to other neurons or target cells. Neurons communicate with each other with chemical neurotransmitters released into a synaptic cleft between two neurons.

Excitatory Versus Inhibitory

One way to classify the synapses is by examining the neurotransmitters' influence on the action potential, either excitatory or inhibitory, in the postsynaptic cell. Once a neurotransmitter crosses the synapse and connects to the neuron's receptor, it has the ability to create an electrical charge that either excites or blocks the receiving neuron. For example, an *excitatory* neurotransmitter triggers an electrical signal that is transmitted down the cell to activate the receiving neuron. In contrast, an *inhibitory* neuron triggers an electrical signal that blocks the signal to the receiving neuron; therefore, a message cannot be carried out.

A neurotransmitter's action can be blocked or removed by three processes: (a) *reuptake*, (b) *degradation*, or (c) *diffusion*, an important step in synaptic transmission. *Reuptake* refers to the process where a neurotransmitter transporter reabsorbs a neurotransmitter after it sends it an impulse or signal. *Degradation* is a process where an enzyme alters the structure of the neurotransmitter so the neurotransmitter is no longer recognized by the receptor. *Diffusion* refers to the process of the neurotransmitter drifting away from the receptor.

Neuron sensitivity of cellular pathways can vary from highly sensitive to less sensitive. This is done by a process known as *cellular modulation* and is important to prevent damage resulting from high concentrations of agonists. *Downregulation* is characterized as an inhibitory response or when available receptors of target cells are suppressed and minimize a response. *Upregulation* refers to the potentiation of a response or an increase in number of receptors available on target cells to generate responses.

Through a process known as *neuroplasticity or neural plasticity* (brain plasticity), the human brain has a remarkable capacity to generate new neuronal connections, adapt, and change throughout the life span to enhance daily functioning. These changes occur in response to genetic, neurobiologic, and environmental influences, along with behaviors, other neural processes, or injury (Wojtalik et al., 2018). These changes in neural pathways and synapses impact the brain's neural functioning. For example, diet, exercise, social interactions, and mindfulness meditation can produce a positive change; on the other hand, stress, a toxic environment, and substance abuse can negatively impact brain functioning. Importantly, neurons differ not only at a functional level, but also at the genomic level and can contribute to behavior and cognitive disorders and other various neurologic diseases.

BASIC PHARMACOLOGIC CONCEPTS

Pharmacology is the study of how drugs affect the body and how the body responds to the drug. Pharmacology includes the drug's chemical properties, biologic effects, and therapeutic uses. *Psychopharmacology* refers to the study of agents derived from natural sources or chemically manufactured in a laboratory that are used to treat psychiatric disorders due to their ability to induce changes in mood, thought, behavior, or sensation. The *bioavailability* refers to the portion of the active form of a drug that reaches systemic circulation or the target site unaltered to employ a biologic response. Bioavailability is a pivotal part of the *pharmacokinetics* paradigm and an essential tool that helps guide individualized dosing regimens. Pharmacokinetics is the study of what the body does to the drug. Pharmacokinetics refers to the timeline of the drug's absorption, bioavailability, distribution, metabolism, and excretion; in other words, the movement of the drug going into, though, and out of the body. *Pharmacodynamics* is the study of what the drug does to the body consistently over the life span: the drug's mechanism of action. How quickly a drug is absorbed determines how quickly it takes effect. The route of administration must be considered when prescribing and dosing medications, because the route of administration directly impacts bioavailability (mouth [PO], intermuscular [IM], intravenous [IV], subcutaneous [SQ], sublingual [SL], per rectum [PR], transdermal) and *population pharmacokinetics*. Population pharmacokinetics enables the analysis of the variability in pharmacokinetics that occurs within and between patients with similar intrinsic characteristics; for example, the variations in drug concentration excreted from patients with renal disease (Dykstra et al., 2015). Additionally, body weight (fat and water weight; lean muscle mass); excretory, hepatic, and renal functioning; serum albumin-level concentration, gastrointestinal motility, metabolic functions, and polypharmacy (e.g., antacids, drug-to-drug interactions); *drug elimination half-life* (the time it takes for 50% of a drug's starting dose to be eliminated); or the presence of other treatments can alter dose concentrations.

Essential Facts

- *Pharmacokinetics* changes throughout the life span.
- *Pharmacodynamics* does not change throughout the life span.

Pharmacogenetics refers to (a) the understanding of how a single heredity gene marker influences one's response to certain medications or (b) how gene variation influences both the pharmacokinetics and pharmacodynamics of a drug. Individual gene variants are applicable to a drug's actions, dose, sensitivity, side effects, and metabolism (Rigter et al., 2020). *Pharmacogenomics* is broader based and relates to all the genes in a genome that may impact a drug's response (Pirmohamed, 2001). The aim of pharmacogenomics is to translate complex genomic information into actionable phenotypes to optimize patient outcomes (Caudle et al., 2018).

DRUG RECEPTOR INTERACTIONS

The cornerstone to psychopharmacology is an understanding of the drug's constant binding action to target receptors. *Affinity* is a term that refers to the drug property that describes its unique ability to bind to the target receptors. Receptors are dormant at rest and are influenced by a drug's ability to turn a signal on or off. Receptors that are switched on can produce biologic responses known as *agonists*. *Antagonists* bind to target receptors; however, antagonists block or switch off the signal. *Partial agonists* bind and activate a receptor but are not able to elicit the greatest possible response that is produced by full agonists. In the presence of a full agonist, a partial agonist will act as an antagonist, competing with the full agonist *for* the same receptor and reduce the ability of the full agonist to generate its maximum effect. *Inverse agonists* bind to receptors and generate the opposite signal from what is expected.

SUMMARY

An understanding of the brain's basic structural regions and the body's sensory and motor system connections to the brain is fundamental to understanding the functional effects of psychotropic drugs. Basic concepts in neurotransmission and general principles of pharmacology have been presented to promote a foundation in understanding the brain and neural structures impacted by psychiatric conditions and to introduce important considerations in prescribing psychotropic medications.

REVIEW QUESTIONS

1. What the drug does to the body is referred to as which one of the following?
   a. Pharmacologic distribution
   b. Pharmacokinetics
   c. Pharmacodynamics
   d. Pharmacoregulation
2. Which one of the answer choices that follow completes this statement? A partial agonist can produce an effect within a cell that ________________.
   a. is not maximal and then blocks the receptor to a full agonist
   b. may bind to the same receptor, but does not produce a response
   c. produces 100% effect within the cell
   d. never binds to a receptor and remains as a free drug
3. The drug property that describes its unique ability to bind to the target receptors is referred to as which one of the following?
   a. Distribution
   b. Affinity
   c. Agonist
   d. Gene transcription
4. The human brain has a remarkable capacity to generate new neuronal connections, adapting and changing throughout the life span to enhance daily functioning. This is referred to as which process?
   a. Neuroplasticity
   b. Antagonism
   c. Transcription
   d. Diffusion
5. A __________ neurotransmitter triggers an electrical signal that is transmitted down the cell and activates the receiving neuron.
   a. Inhibitory
   b. Dominant
   c. Excitatory
   d. Modulatory

REFERENCES

Baumann, O., Borra, R. J., Bower, J. M., Cullen, K. E., Habas, C., Ivry, R. B., Leggio, M., Mattingley, J. B., Molinari, M., Moulton, E. A., Paulin, M. G., Pavlova, M. A., Schmahmann, J. D., & Sokolov, A. A. (2015). Consensus paper: The role of the cerebellum in perceptual processes. *Cerebellum*, *14*(2), 197–220. https://doi.org/10.1007/s12311-014-0627-7

Braslow, J., & Marder, S. (2019). History of psychopharmacology. *Annual Review of Clinical Psychology*, *15*, 25–50. https://doi.org/10.1146/annurev-clinpsy-050718-095514

Caudle, K. E., Keeling, N. J., Klein, T. E., Whirl-Carrillo, M., Pratt, V. M., & Hoffman, J. M. (2018). Standardization can accelerate the adoption of pharmacogenomics: Current status and the path forward. *Pharmacogenomics*, *19*(10), 847–860. https://doi.org/10.2217/pgs-2018-0028

Dykstra, K., Mehrotra, N., Tornøe, C. W., Kastrissios, H., Patel, B., Al-Huniti, N., Jadhav, P., Wang, Y., & Byon, W. (2015). Reporting guidelines for population pharmacokinetic analyses. *Journal of Pharmacokinetics and Pharmacodynamics*, *42*(3), 301–314. https://doi.org/10.1007/s10928-015-9417-1

Pirmohamed, M. (2001). Pharmacogenetics and pharmacogenomics. *British Journal of Clinical Pharmacology*, *52*(4), 345–347. https://doi.org/10.1046/j.0306-5251.2001.01498.x

Rigter, T., Jansen, M. E., de Groot, J. M., Janssen, S., Rodenburg, W., & Cornel, M. C. (2020). Implementation of pharmacogenetics in primary care: A multi-stakeholder perspective. *Frontiers in Genetics*, *11*, Article 10. https://doi.org/10.3389/fgene.2020.00010

Shin, M., Wang, Y., Borgus, J. R., & Venton, B. J. (2019). Electrochemistry at the synapse. *Annual Review of Analytical Chemistry*, *12*(1), 297–321. https://doi.org/10.1146/annurev-anchem-061318-115434

Wojtalik, J. A., Eack, S. M., Smith, M. J., & Keshavan, M. S. (2018). Using cognitive neuroscience to improve mental health treatment: A comprehensive review. *Journal of the Society for Social Work and Research*, *9*(2), 223–260. https://doi.org/10.1086/697566

4

Neurotransmitters Overview

Neurotransmitters are endogenous chemicals that enable communication between neurons. Specifically, neurotransmitters are the brain chemicals that help relay messages from one part of the brain to another and between the brain and the rest of the body, primarily through synaptic transmission, also referred to as neurotransmission. The signals sent by neurotransmitters are responsible for the vast majority of brain and motor functions, including memory, planning, heart rate, respirations, digestion, hormonal responses, movement, and others. Many different diseases involve increased or decreased levels of neurotransmitters in the brain, which lead to different clinical features. Understanding the role of neurotransmitters and receptors in the brain is essential to gain insights into the neural bases of critical brain functions and pathologic conditions, such as anxiety, depression, schizophrenia, Parkinson's disease, drug addiction, learning problems, and many more. This chapter will provide an overview of (a) the different types of neurotransmitters and their functions, (b) the fundamental mechanisms of neuronal excitability, (c) signal generation and transmission, (d) synaptic transmission, (e) neural plasticity, (f) different types of receptors, and (g) the different illnesses and medications that target these receptors.

In this chapter you will learn:

1. To understand the various functions of neurotransmitters
2. To describe neurotransmission processes in the brain and nervous system
3. To differentiate the actions of excitatory and inhibitory neurotransmitters

4. To comprehend the neural bases of critical brain functions and pathologic conditions
5. To understand the role of neurotransmitters in behavior and cognition

NEUROTRANSMISSION

Dopamine System

Dopamine plays a vital role in the brain's reward system by helping to reinforce certain behaviors via rewards or pleasurable sensations. Dopamine is often referred to as the "feel good" or "pleasure" neurotransmitter and is the most extensively studied neurotransmitter. Dopamine is classified as a *catecholamine* that is fundamental to the maintenance of homeostasis through the autonomic nervous system. Catecholamines are produced in the brain, adrenal glands, and nerve tissue and function as both neurotransmitters and hormones. Dopamine is a derivative of the amino acid tyrosine and is primarily produced in the *substantia nigra, ventral tegmental area* (VTA), and *hypothalamus.* The five dopaminergic receptor subtypes are referred to as D_1, D_2, D_3, D_4, and D_5. Dopamine is involved in the central nervous system, digestion, and in renal, motor, and cognitive functions. Additionally, dopamine is responsible for uplifting mood, motivation, and alertness, and is a critical modulator for learning, emotional responses, blood vessel tone, psychosis, and prolactin inhibition. Primary conditions associated with dopamine include schizophrenia, Parkinson's disease, attention deficit hyperactivity disorder (ADHD), and drug addiction.

Essential Facts

Dopaminergic Receptor Subtypes

- D_1: memory, attentiveness, impulse control, motor activity regulation, renal function
- D_2: motor activity, attentiveness, sleep, memory, learning
- D_3: cognition, impulse control, attentiveness, sleep
- D_4: cognition, impulse control, attentiveness, sleep
- D_5: decision-making, cognition, attentiveness, renin secretion
- D_1 and D_5 receptors activate adenylyl cyclase
- D_2 through D_4 receptors inhibit adenylyl cyclase

There are eight dopaminergic pathways. The four major pathways are the mesolimbic pathway, the mesocortical pathway, the nigrostriatal pathway, and the tuberoinfundibular pathway. The mesolimbic pathway begins dopamine transport from the VTA to the nucleus accumbens. This pathway is responsible for dopamine's pleasure and reward functions along with memory and motivating behaviors.

Essential Facts

In the Greek language, the word *meso* means "middle." The prefix "meso" in the word *mesolimbic* refers to the midbrain or "middle brain."

Essential Facts

The Reward Network

- Ventral tegmental area
- Nucleus accumbens
- Prefrontal cortex (anterior cingulate ventral cortex)
- Amygdala
- Hippocampus

Additionally, due to projections that innervate other regions of the forebrain, the mesolimbic pathway contributes to the positive symptoms of schizophrenia. Blocking the mesolimbic pathway with antipsychotic medications reduces intense emotions, hallucinations, delusions, and thought disorganization. The mesocortical pathway—a dopaminergic pathway that connects the ventral tegmentum to the prefrontal cortex—is the part of the brain highly involved in cognition, working memory, and decision-making. The negative symptoms associated with schizophrenia, such as apathy, flat affect, alogia, avolition, and cognitive impairments, are associated with malfunctions of the mesocortical pathway and the dorsolateral prefrontal cortex.

Essential Facts

Dopaminergic Pathways Relevant to Antipsychotics in the Treatment of Schizophrenia

- Mesolimbic pathway: positive symptoms
- Mesocortical pathway: negative symptoms
- Nigrostriatal pathway: extrapyramidal symptoms and tardive dyskinesia
- Tuberoinfundibular pathway: hyperprolactinemia

The nigrostriatal pathway transports dopamine from the subtantia nigra to the dorsal striatum (caudate nucleus and putamen) in the forebrain. The main function of this pathway is to influence voluntary movement and motor planning. Parkinson's disease is associated with loss of nigrostriatal dopaminergic innervation. The clinical features associated with Parkinson's disease (tremor, rigidity, bradykinesia, and postural instability) are associated with dopaminergic receptor malfunction within the nigrostriatal pathway.

The tuberoinfundibular pathway is characterized as the process of transmitting a bundle of dopamine neurons from the hypothalamus to the pituitary gland to influence prolactin secretion. The major role of the D_2 receptor in the pituitary gland is to inhibit the synthesis and secretion of prolactin; however, hyperprolactinemia occurs when antipsychotic medications block dopamine receptors in this pathway.

Essential Facts

- Antipsychotic drugs block the D_2 receptor.
- Compared to typical antipsychotics, atypical antipsychotics bind loosely to dopamine D_2 receptors to decrease dopamine availability.
- For example, treatment for schizophrenia includes medications that aim to lower dopamine availability; however, Parkinson's disease includes medications that aim to increase dopamine availability; these medications are referred to as dopamine receptor agonists.
- Improper levels of dopamine in certain regions of the brain are associated with schizophrenia, drug addiction, psychosis, depression, Tourette syndrome, and attention deficit hyperactivity disorder (ADHD).
- Dopamine-related neurodegenerative diseases include Parkinson's disease, multiple sclerosis, and Huntington's disease.

SEROTONIN

Serotonin (5-hydroxytryptamine [5-HT]), a complex neurotransmitter that is part of the monoaminergic neurotransmitter system, sends signals between nerve cells in the brain to influence myriad brain and body functions. Serotonin gets its name from its origin, the serum, and its ability to increase tone or vasoconstriction, hence the name "sero-tonin" (Terry & Margolis, 2017).

Serotonin exhibits both excitatory and inhibitory neurotransmission and influences a variety of important functions, such as mood, sleep, cognition, digestion, and sexual functioning. Serotonin also promotes platelet binding, bone formation (osteoporosis), appetite, and memory. Additionally, serotonin is linked to the peristaltic reflex and the stimulation of intestinal propulsion (Mawe & Hoffman, 2013; Terry & Margolis, 2017). Serotonin imbalances in certain brain regions along with faulty intracellular pathway signaling is postulated to be responsible for mood regulation and impulsivity and is central to the pathophysiology of depression. Although serotonin has been studied for over 70 years and there is evidence that serotonin is involved in mood regulation, exactly how remains obscure, and no unified consensus exists (Bektaş et al., 2020; Terry & Margolis, 2017).

Serotonin is produced in different areas of the body. Ninety percent of the total serotonin in the body is produced, stored, and released from a subset of enteroendocrine cells called enterochromaffin that are located inside the gastrointestinal tract. Approximately 1% to 2% of the total amount of serotonin in the body is made by serotonergic neurons in the brain (Bektaş et al., 2020). 5-HT comes from the *raphe nuclei*, a cluster of nuclei situated in the brainstem throughout the midbrain, pons, and medulla. L-Tryptophan, supplied by dietary protein, is the precursor amino acid required for synthesis of serotonin production. Serotonin is most abundant in the cerebral cortex (hippocampal region) and the ventromedial prefrontal cortex. Serotonin can be excitatory in the raphe nucleus and inhibitory in the cerebral cortex.

Essential Facts

Monoamine Action

- Acetylcholine: excitatory
- Dopamine: primarily inhibitory
- Gamma aminobutyric acid (GABA): inhibitory
- Glutamate: excitatory
- Norepinephrine: primarily excitatory but can be inhibitory
- Serotonin: excitatory raphe nuclei and inhibitory in the cerebral cortex

Most 5-HT receptors are postsynaptic, with the exception of 5-HT1A and 5-HT1B, which are primarily presynaptic and regulate 5-HT release (Virk et al., 2016). The discovery of additional receptor subtypes for 5-HT made it necessary to establish a system of unambiguous nomenclature based on 5-HT's operational qualities, drug-related features, and other characteristics. To understand 5-HT receptor regulation, it is first critical to understand the messenger systems, intricate pathways and linkages, and roots of neural pathophysiology underlying disease etiology.

Essential Facts

The monoamine hypothesis suggests that the basis of depression is a reduction in the levels of serotonin (5-HT), dopamine, and norepinephrine in the body.

Essential Facts

Functions of Serotonin in the Brain and Body

- Anxiety and stress
- Depression and mood
- Impulsivity and aggression

(*continued*)

Essential Facts (*continued*)

- Learning and cognition
- Nausea
- Obsessions and compulsions
- Pain and headaches
- Platelet binding
- Sexual functioning

Serotonin Syndrome

Serotonin syndrome is a medication-induced condition resulting from serotonergic overactivity at the synapses of the central and peripheral nervous systems, with the most common drug triggers being antidepressants. Serotonin syndrome occurs when serotonergic medications are combined with other selective serotonin reuptake inhibitors, monoamine oxidase inhibitors, tricyclic antidepressants, and other medications that increase serotonin levels to dangerously high levels.

Even though it is uncommon, serotonin syndrome is a potentially life-threatening condition that can be challenging to diagnose. No laboratory tests can reliably diagnose serotonin syndrome; therefore, diagnosis is made by presenting clinical features and a review of current medications. Furthermore, signs and symptoms of serotonin syndrome can vary in severity. The diagnostic basis of serotonin syndrome includes the triad of altered mental status, autonomic hyperactivity, and neuromuscular abnormalities.

Essential Facts

Symptoms of Serotonin Syndrome

- Agitation
- Akathisia
- Clonus
- Coma
- Confusion
- Diaphoresis
- Diarrhea
- Hyperactive bowel sounds
- Hypertension
- Hyperreflexia
- Hyperthermia
- Hypervigilance
- Hypomania

(*continued*)

Essential Facts (*continued*)

- Loss of coordination
- Myoclonus
- Mydriasis
- Rigidity
- Seizures
- Sweating
- Tachycardia
- Tremors

NOREPINEPHRINE

Norepinephrine, or noradrenaline, structured as a catecholamine, functions as both a neurotransmitter and a stress hormone and is vital to the central and sympathetic nervous systems. Norepinephrine is released from noradrenergic neurons originating from the *locus coeruleus*, the primary source of norepinephrine production (Rodenkirch et al., 2019). Norepinephrine neurons project to all areas of the central nervous system to modulate various behavioral and physiologic processes and have been linked to focused attention, distractibility, mood, arousal, sleep, memory, appetite, and homeostasis (Dahl et al., 2020; Robertson et al., 2013).

Within the sympathetic nervous system, norepinephrine is fundamental to the flight-or-fight response due to its ability to bind to certain adrenergic receptors. There are two subtypes of receptors: (a) alpha-adrenergic receptors (α), which are primarily responsible for smooth muscle contraction, and (b) beta-adrenergic receptors (β), which are primarily responsible for smooth muscle relaxation. These receptors are divided into subtypes: (a) α-1 and α-2 and (b) β-1, β-2, and β-3.

α-1 receptors trigger the release of calcium from calcium storage structures, which influences muscle contractility. α-1 receptors are key to the body's sympathetic nervous system's fight-or-flight response because they activate smooth muscle contraction, such as vasoconstriction and pupil dilation. In contrast, α-2 is an inhibitory neurotransmitter mainly located on peripheral presynaptic nerve terminals. α-2 is part of the negative feedback system because, when these receptors are activated, lower levels of norepinephrine are released, and the sympathetic nervous system is deactivated. Notably, α-2 receptors are also located on platelets. When activated, α-2 releases platelets to promote platelet aggregation.

β-1 receptors are located on the heart and increase heart rate when activated. β-2 receptors are mainly located on the lungs, gastrointestinal tract, and blood vessels. When activated, β-2s produce smooth muscle relaxation. Lastly, β-3 receptors are primarily located in adipose tissue, which is less clinically relevant in psychiatry.

Essential Facts

Adrenergic Receptors Summary

- α-1: contracts smooth muscle
- α-2: presynaptic nerve terminal
- β-1: heart and kidney
- β-2: relaxes smooth muscle, eyes
- β-3: adipose tissue

GAMMA-AMINOBUTYRIC ACID

Gamma-aminobutyric acid (GABA) is a nonprotein amino acid that is present throughout various brain regions. GABA synthesis occurs via the α-decarboxylation of l-glutamate by the enzyme glutamic acid decarboxylase. Commonly referred to as the central nervous system's major inhibitory neurotransmitter, GABA serves as a mediator to regulate the glutamanergic excitatory counterpart. Its physiologic roles are associated with the modulation of synaptic transmission, promotion of calmness and relaxation, and prevention of sleeplessness. In addition to GABA's role in the body's stress response, it also plays an important role in behavior and cognition, such as impulsivity and risky decision-making. For example, deficits in GABA are associated with drug and alcohol addiction, obsessive-compulsive disorder, and ADHD. GABA is divided into two distinct classes of receptors: $GABA_A$ and $GABA_B$ (Ngo & Vo, 2019). $GABA_A$ is more prominent in the brain and associated with psychotropic agents such as benzodiazepines, ethanol, and barbiturates (Ngo & Vo, 2019).

Essential Facts

Glutamate and GABA neurons and receptors are located in the hypothalamus, where they regulate neurohormone release, circadian activity, and other hypothalamic functions (Belousov et al., 2001).

GLUTAMATE

Glutamate is the major mediator of excitatory signals and is considered to be the most dominant neurotransmitter in neural circuit communication in the brain and central nervous system. As an excitatory neurotransmitter, glutamate has a high propensity to activate neurons or potentiate action potentials within neural circuits. Within the brain, glutaminase synthesizes glutamine into glutamate. Glutamate plays an essential role in normal brain functioning. In the cortex and hippocampus, glutamate impacts learning and memory, sensory inputs, motor coordination, and emotional responses, and has been linked to the activity of most other neurotransmitter systems.

Glutamate receptors are abundant throughout the central nervous system and are also located in *glial cells.* Glial cells are responsible for modulating extracellular glutamate levels because tight regulation of extracellular glutamate concentrations is critical for normal synaptic transmission and to prevent *neuronal hyperexcitability*, also referred to as *excitotoxicity* or *glutamatergic storm,* which, if sustained, causes cell death. Activation of a presynaptic neuron causes the release of glutamate, which then binds to postsynaptic glutamate ionotropic receptors *N*-methyl *D*-aspartate (NMDA) and α-amino-3-hydroxy-5-methyl-4-isoxazolepropionic acid (AMPA), which are Kainite receptors. Notably, modulating glutamate also has neuroprotective properties. Glutamate can release neurotrophic factors, including brain-derived neurotrophic factors, or BDNF, which help to grow new neurons and synapses and support existing neurons.

Essential Facts

- Synaptic plasticity is the brain's ability to strengthen neural connections required for signal transferring between neurons.
- The term *glia* is from the Greek word meaning "glue" to reflect the belief that glia cells held the nervous system together.

ACETYLCHOLINE

Acetylcholine (ACh), a neurotransmitter made of choline and acetyl coenzyme A (AcCoA), is an essential neurotransmitter in both the central and peripheral nervous systems. ACh is located in the nucleus basalis of the Meynert in the substantia innominata of the forebrain. ACh controls the sympathetic and parasympathetic branches of the autonomous nervous system to mediate the "rest and digest" function, where the parasympathetic system is mediated by *muscarinic receptors* in peripheral organs to conserve energy by slowing heart rate, increasing intestinal and gland activity, emptying the bladder, moderating gland secretion and pupillary constriction, and relaxing sphincter tone in the gastrointestinal tract (Naser & Kuner, 2018). In other words, the sympathetic nervous system prepares the body for fight-or-flight. The parasympathetic nervous system functions as the unconscious energy-conserving system.

Two classes of cholinergic receptors respond to ACh: (a) muscarinic receptors, which function in both the peripheral nervous system and CNS, and (b) nicotinic receptors, which function within the CNS and neuromuscular junction. At the neuromuscular junction, nicotinic receptors function to convey the signal of voluntary movement. Nicotinic receptors on ACh are also located in the brain's reward pathway and are hypothesized to underlie nicotine's addictive properties. The drug varenicline (Chantix) is used to inhibit nicotine's reward action. In the hippocampus, amygdala, and cerebral cortex, nicotinic receptors are involved with cognitive processes, including attention, long-term memory, working memory, and memory formation to consolidation and retrieval in memory formation. Degeneration of cholinergic neurons such as ACh impacts both the peripheral and central nervous systems and plays a role in the development of Alzheimer's disease, Parkinson's disease, schizophrenia, epilepsy, and addiction. Drugs that increase ACh levels in the brain are used in patients with Alzheimer's disease. Malfunctions within neuromuscular junctions are seen in neurologic disorders such as myasthenia gravis and other congenital myasthenic syndromes.

Essential Facts

The autonomic nervous system, divided into sympathetic and parasympathetic divisions, maintains the body's homeostatic environment by adjusting neuronal, circulatory, respiratory, integumentary, digestive, and urinary systems.

HISTAMINE

Histamine is a monoamine that induces excitatory signals to target neurons. In the periphery, histamine is often linked to mast cells, the immune system, and gastric secretions. In the central nervous system, histamine has been linked in psychiatric diseases. Histamine synthesis takes place in both the posterior basal hypothalamus and the tuberomammillary nucleus (TMN), and sends signals throughout the central nervous system (Sheffler & Reddy, n.d.). Many transmitter systems interact with histaminergic neurons in the brain and function to (a) promote wakefulness and thermoregulation, (b) modulate food and water intake and endocrine functions (regulates hypothalamic functions), and (c) reduce seizure activity and decrease motivational behavior (Scammell et al., 2019). There are four distinct G protein-coupled histamine receptors: H1, H2, H3, and H4 (H1R–H4R).

Essential Facts

- Signaling through the H1 receptor promotes arousal; therefore, drugs that block the H1 receptor are commonly used for insomnia. Other H1 blockers used for insomnia include antidepressants and antipsychotics, such as doxepin, amitriptyline, and olanzapine.
- H3-receptor inverse agonists such as pitolisant promote wakefulness.

(*continued*)

Essential Facts (*continued*)

The roles of histamine include the following:

- Arousal or wake-promoting effects
- Gastric secretion production
- Mediation of aggressive, anxiety, and panic behavior
- Rapid eye movement
- Release of ACh, dopamine, norepinephrine, serotonin
- Vasodilation

OPIOID RECEPTORS

Opioids are analgesics and euphoriants that, in high doses, can cause sedation and respiratory depression. The action of opioid compounds is mediated through activation of specific opioid receptors. There are three main opioid receptors in the central nervous system—delta, kappa, and mu—in areas associated with pain perception. Mu opioid receptors are linked to mood, pain, and reward. Delta opioid receptors are associated with mood. Kappa receptors impact mood, reward, analgesia, dysphoria, and increases in urination. Within the peripheral organs, opioid receptors are located in the heart, lungs, liver, and gastrointestinal and reproductive tracts.

SUMMARY

The brain is a fragile neuronal organ system. It is important to understand how altered monoamine signaling is associated with mental health conditions. Neurotransmission is the transferring of a signal from a sending neuron to a receiving neuron across the synapse. These signals are responsible for most of the brain and motor functions and can impact mood and behavior. Clinicians need to be vigilant of patients taking high-risk medication(s) that may result in serotonin syndrome. Serotonin syndrome is a medication-induced clinical condition resulting from serotonergic hyperactivity, and has been linked to a variety of drugs with direct and indirect serotonergic actions; symptoms can range from mild and self-limiting to life threatening.

REVIEW QUESTIONS

1. Drugs that increase __________ levels in the brain are used in patients with Alzheimer's disease.
   a. Serotonin
   b. Dopamine
   c. Acetylcholine
   d. Norepinephrine

2. Which one of the following receptors on acetylcholine is also located in the brain's reward pathway and is hypothesized to underlie nicotine's addictive properties?
   a. Histaminergic
   b. Norepinephrine
   c. Serotonergic receptors
   d. Nicotinic receptors
3. Which one of the following statements best describes glutamate?
   a. Glutamate is the major mediator of excitatory signals in neurotransmission.
   b. Glutamate is a recessive inhibitory neurotransmitter.
   c. Glutamate is the major regulator of the inhibitory mu receptor site.
   d. Glutamate is the major mediator of inhibitory transmitter in the brain.
4. GABA plays an important role in behavior and cognition, involving actions such as which one of the following?
   a. Impulsivity and risky decision-making
   b. Laughter and visualization
   c. Fear and trust
   d. Brain protection and growth
5. Mu opioid receptors are linked to which one of the following?
   a. Mood, pain, and reward
   b. Analgesia and increases in urination
   c. Dysphoria and excessive daytime sleepiness
   d. Arousal and impulsivity

REFERENCES

Bektaş, A., Erdal, H., Ulusoy, M., & Uzbay, I. T. (2020). Does serotonin in the intestines make you happy? *Turkish Journal of Gastroenterology, 31*(10), 721–723. https://doi.org/10.5152/tjg.2020.19554

Belousov, A. B., O'Hara, B. F., & Denisova, J. V. (2001). Acetylcholine becomes the major excitatory neurotransmitter in the hypothalamus in vitro in the absence of glutamate excitation. *Journal of Neuroscience, 21*(6), 2015–2027. https://doi.org/10.1523/JNEUROSCI.21-06-02015.2001

Dahl, M. J., Mather, M., Sander, M. C., & Werkle-Bergner, M. (2020). Noradrenergic responsiveness supports selective attention across the adult lifespan. *Journal of Neuroscience, 40*(22), 4372–4390. https://doi.org/10.1523/JNEUROSCI.0398-19.2020

Mawe, G. M., & Hoffman, J. M. (2013). Serotonin signaling in the gut–functions, dysfunctions and therapeutic targets. *Nature Reviews: Gastroenterology & Hepatology, 10*(8), 473–486. https://doi.org/10.1038/nrgastro.2013.105

Naser, P. V., & Kuner, R. (2018). Molecular, cellular and circuit basis of cholinergic modulation of pain. *Neuroscience, 387*, 135–148. https://doi.org/10.1016/j.neuroscience.2017.08.049

Ngo, D. H., & Vo, T. S. (2019). An updated review on pharmaceutical properties of gamma-aminobutyric acid. *Molecules, 24*(15), Article 2678. https://doi.org/10.3390/molecules24152678

Robertson, S. D., Plummer, N. W., de Marchena, J., & Jensen, P. (2013). Developmental origins of central norepinephrine neuron diversity. *Nature Neuroscience, 16*(8), 1016–1023. https://doi.org/10.1038/nn.3458

Rodenkirch, C., Liu, Y., Schriver, B. J., & Wang, Q. (2019). Locus coeruleus activation enhances thalamic feature selectivity via norepinephrine regulation of intrathalamic circuit dynamics. *Nature Neuroscience*, *22*(1), 120–133. https://doi.org/10.1038/s41593-018-0283-1

Scammell, T. E., Jackson, A. C., Franks, N. P., Wisden, W., & Dauvilliers, Y. (2019). Histamine: Neural circuits and new medications. *Sleep*, *42*(1), Article zsy183. https://doi.org/10.1093/sleep/zsy183

Sheffler, Z., Reddy, V. (2022, May 8). Physiology, neurotransmitters. StatPearls. Accessed September 1, 2022 from https://www.ncbi.nlm.nih.gov/books/NBK539894/

Terry, N., & Margolis, K. G. (2017). Serotonergic mechanisms regulating the GI tract: Experimental evidence and therapeutic relevance. In Greenwood-Van Meerveld. B. (Ed.), *Handbook of experimental pharmacology* (Vol. 239, pp. 319–342). Springer.

Virk, M. S., Sagi, Y., Medrihan, L., Leung, J., Kaplitt, M. G., & Greengard, P. (2016). Opposing roles for serotonin in cholinergic neurons of the ventral and dorsal striatum. *Proceedings of the National Academy of Sciences of the United States of America*, *113*(3), 734–739. https://doi.org/10.1073/pnas.1524183113

II

Major Classes of Psychiatric Medications

5

Antidepressants

Major depressive disorder (MDD) is one of the most common unipolar affective disorders for individuals of all ages and is associated with hypofunction of the serotonergic system. Although there is no consensus regarding the cause of depression, theories such as the monoamine theory or the neurotransmitter hypothesis contribute to scientists' understanding of depression. These theories discuss imbalances of serotonin, dopamine, and norepinephrine and other modulating neurohormones. More contemporary theories consider depression to be a clinically heterogeneous disorder because depression originates from genetic, biochemical, and environmental factors. Depression rates increase from childhood through adolescence and into adulthood. Early recognition and intervention are the key to treatment. Treatment for depression includes psychotherapy and antidepressant medications to minimize clinical morbidity and improve clinical outcomes. Although the risk of suicidality may increase upon initiation of antidepressants, suicide risk also increases with untreated depression; therefore, careful consideration is required when managing depressed individuals (Gautam et al., 2017). This chapter details medications for the treatment of MDD.

In this chapter you will learn:

1. How to compare pharmacologic options for depression
2. How to name five or more criteria for major depressive disorder (MDD)
3. How to identify screening tools for MDD
4. How to evaluate medication safety considerations in depression management
5. How to assess therapeutic responses in depressed patients

SIMPLIFIED DIAGNOSTIC CRITERIA FOR DEPRESSION

To meet the criterion for MDD, individuals must experience five or more of the listed symptoms during a two-week period with at least one of the symptoms being (a) depressed mood or (b) anhedonia or reduced ability to experience pleasure. To diagnose depression, the symptoms must cause significant distress or impairment in social, occupational, or other important areas of functioning. Substance use or another medical condition must not be causing any of the symptoms (American Psychiatric Association, 2013). The criteria for MDD are as follows:

1. Depressed mood, bleak and pessimistic views of the future (in children, irritable mood)
2. Anhedonia or reduced ability to experience pleasure, or diminished interest in activities
3. Weight loss or weight gain when not dieting or experiencing changes in appetite
4. Slowing down of thought and decreases of physical movement
5. Fatigue or loss of energy
6. Ideas of unworthiness, reduced self-esteem, poor self-confidence, and guilt
7. Difficulties in thought processes, difficulty with concentration, or indecisiveness
8. Ideas or acts of self-harm, recurrent suicidal ideation without a plan, a suicide attempt, or a detailed plan for suicide

Essential Facts

Children under 18 years old often present with more somatic complaints, irritableness, symptoms of anxiety, trouble verbalizing feelings, marked decreased interest in play, self-destructive themes in play, thoughts of unworthiness or suicide, crying or shouting outbursts, observed anhedonia, low self-esteem, guilt, hopelessness, increased boredom, decreased grades, and poor school performance. Symptoms do not need to be present for two weeks.

DEPRESSIVE DISORDERS

Table 5.1 lists the American Psychiatric Association ([APA] 2013) depressive disorders and key features.

SCREENING TOOLS

Since there are no laboratory tests specific to depression, depression screening using reliable and valid instruments can be used for detecting the presence or absence of symptoms; making a formal diagnosis; assessing of changes in symptom severity; and monitoring client outcomes.

Table 5.1

Depression-Related Disorders

Disorder	Key Features
MDD, single episode or recurrent episode	Depression symptoms that occur most of the day, nearly every day, and may include persistent low mood, sadness, tearfulness, emptiness or hopelessness, irritability or frustration, loss of interest or pleasure, low self-esteem and self-confidence compared to usual for the individual, feelings of guilt, decreased mental and physical energy, slowed thinking, speaking or body movements, sleep disturbances, changes in weight and appetite, anxiety, agitation or restlessness, recurrent thoughts of death, suicidal thoughts, suicide attempts or suicide, unexplained somatic complaints that are severe enough to affect the overall quality of life and functioning
Persistent depressive disorder (dysthymia)	At least 2 years (adults) or 1 year (children and adolescents) of depressed mood, most of the day, for most days, with impaired ability to experience pleasure, and other depressive symptoms (sleep, appetite, low energy, etc.) severe enough to affect the overall quality of life and functioning
Disruptive mood dysregulation disorder (DMDD)	Diagnosed in children (before age 10, and the diagnosis should not be made for the first time before age 6 or after age 18) who present with recurrent irritable or angry mood (most of the day, on most days) and severe temper outbursts (three or more per week) for at least 12 months, with no more than 3 or fewer months without meeting criteria in two or more settings at home, in school, or with peers and that interfere with their functioning
Premenstrual dysphoric disorder (PMDD)	For 1 year, for most menstrual cycles, mood lability, irritability, anxiety, tension, tearful, angry, depressed mood, low energy, as well as decreased interest in activities, physical symptoms such as breast tenderness, abdominal bloating, sleep, appetite, and so on, that occur in the luteal phase of the menstrual cycle and resolve within a few days of onset of menses and improve within a few days after the onset of menses
Substance/medication-induced depressive disorder	Evidence from history, lab findings, or physical exam; a depressed mood or diminished interest in most activities that occurred during or after exposure to an underlying substance or medication
Depressive disorder due to another medical condition	Persistent depressed mood symptoms that are reflective of an underlying medical condition and not better explained by another mental condition
Other specified depressive disorder	Depressive symptoms causing distress and social and occupational impairments but do not meet the full criteria for any of the disorders in the depressive disorders diagnostic class.
Unspecified depressive disorder	Characteristic of a depressive disorder that causes distress but there is insufficient information to make a more specific diagnosis

PEDIATRIC SCREENING TOOLS

- Beck Depression Inventory for Primary Care (BDI-PC)
- Center for Epidemiologic Studies Depression Scale for Children (CES-DC)

- Children's Depression Inventory (CDI)
- Children's Depression Scale (CDS)
- Mood Feeling Questionnaire (MFQ)
- Patient Health Questionnaire Modified for Adolescents (PHQ-A)

ADULT AND OLDER ADULTS SCREENING TOOLS

- Beck Depression Inventory (BDI or BDI-II)
- Center for Epidemiologic Studies Depression Scale (CES-D)
- Depression Scale (DEPS)
- Duke Anxiety-Depression Scale (DADS)
- Geriatric Depression Scale (GDS)
- Inventory of Depressive Symptomatology—Clinician Rated (IDS-C)
- Montgomery Asberg Depression Rating Scale
- Mood Disorder Questionnaire (MDQ)
- Patient Health Questionnaire (PHQ-2 and PHQ-9)
- Symptom Check-List-90 Revised (SCL-90-R)

Essential Facts

Assessing for Mood and Anhedonia

- In the past 2 weeks, have you been bothered by having little interest or pleasure in doing things?
- In the past 2 weeks, have you been feeling down, depressed, or hopeless?

An answer of "yes" to either question requires a more in-depth assessment. (Lam et al., 2016)

CLINICAL PRESENTATION FOR OLDER ADULTS WITH DEPRESSION

Often, older adults do not report a depressed mood, but instead present with less specific symptoms such as fatigue, insomnia, anorexia, and treatment-resistant pain symptoms. Older adults may also dismiss less mild depression as a normal part of aging or an appropriate response to expected life stressors. Other features that may suggest depression include the following:

- Fatigue
- Frequent office visits or use of medical services
- Headache
- Increased dependency
- Insistent reports of pain

- Insomnia
- Sleep or appetite changes
- Social isolation
- Unexplained gastrointestinal symptoms

Essential Facts

Although not diagnostic, the MDQ, a 17-question screening tool, can be helpful when differentiating between unipolar depression and bipolar depression.

MANAGEMENT CONSIDERATIONS

Management of depression involves comprehensive assessment based on a detailed patient history, collateral sources, physical examination, and mental state examinations to properly establish diagnosis. Depression can also be caused by organic or medication-induced etiology. Management options for MDD in children, adolescents, and adults vary in severity. Mild to moderate depression may be managed with psychoeducation, family education, and psychotherapy, whereas more severe depressive episodes may require pharmacotherapy.

Essential Facts

Organic Etiologies for Depressive States

- Thyroid-stimulating hormone dysfunction
- Nutritional deficiencies
- Iron studies
- Blood glucose levels

In general, because of their side effects and safety profile, selective serotonin reuptake inhibitors (SSRIs) are the firstline antidepressant agents. Considerations for the type of SSRI include the following:

- Adverse effect profile
- Availability and cost
- Comorbidities
- Danger of overdose
- Past treatment response (personal and family) or side effects
- Patient and guardian preference
- Possible drug interactions
- Severity of the patient's depression
- Timing of therapeutic effect

Medications should not be the only form of treatment for depressed patients; instead, medication should be used in combination with psychotherapy. It is important to note that informed consent is an ongoing process; discussions of therapeutic options must include the risks, benefits, alternative management options, clear goals, and expectations for treatment, along with an opportunity for the patient to ask questions. Providers must also assess for social support, stigma, personal coping, and caregiver burden. A thorough review of the patient's diagnosis, possible underlying conditions and issues, patient adherence, patient pharmacokinetic and pharmacodynamic factors, and the patient's treatment plan must be conducted after 4 to 8 weeks of treatment if no improvement is observed.

It is important to recognize that somatic complaints and psychologic symptoms of depression can co-occur, mimic depressive symptoms, or coexist; therefore, contributing medical diagnoses is an essential consideration in the assessment of patients who present with depressive symptomatology.

LAB MONITORING CONSIDERATIONS

Blood Pressure

- Baseline, 1 month, and with dose changes

Bone Mineral Density

- Baseline in older adults and follow-up as clinically indicated

Electrocardiogram (EKG)

- Baseline and dose changes
- Monitor children and older adults with more caution

Body Mass Index (BMI)

- Baseline, repeat 4 to 6 weeks and 6 months

Electrolytes

- Baseline, repeat 4 to 6 weeks and 6 months
- Monitor older adults for hyponatremia with more caution
- Assess fall risk due to hypotension

Pregnancy Test

- If applicable

Screen for Prevalence of Potentially Inappropriate Medication (PIM) in Older Adults

- Associated with increased morbidity, mortality, and decrease in quality of life
- Screening Tool in Older Persons' Prescriptions (STOPP)
- Beers Criteria

Suicidality

- Baseline, daily, weekly, monthly, or variable depending on clinical presentation

Thyroid Tests

- Baseline and follow-up as clinically indicated

Vitamin D, B_{12}, Folate

- Baseline and if clinically indicated

HIGH-RISK GROUPS FOR DEPRESSION

- Family history of depression
- Individuals with other psychiatric disorders
- Lower socioeconomic status
- Personal history of chronic medical diseases
- Substance misuse
- Unemployed
- Women

Essential Facts

Fluoxetine may be more favorable for an individual with a history of intermittent missed doses due to its longer half-life; however, fluoxetine takes longer to achieve steady therapeutic states compared to other antidepressant medications (Mullen, 2018).

Essential Facts

- When prescribing antidepressant medications, consider the drug's relative toxicity or safety in overdose. For example, fatal overdose profile is lower with SSRIs than with tricyclic antidepressants.
- Start antidepressant on low dose to assess tolerability, then titrate upward to assess efficacy.

GENERAL SELECTIVE SEROTONIN REUPTAKE INHIBITOR PRESCRIBING CONSIDERATIONS FOR CHILDREN AND ADOLESCENTS

- Adjust based on benefits-to-risk ratio optimization
- Note they may activate bipolar disorder and suicidal ideation

- Assess growth (height and weight)
- If no response in 4 to 6 weeks, consider alternative medication and/or reassess diagnosis
- Assess for activation, restlessness, jitteriness, hyperactivity, hypomania, or mania
- Note increased risk for suicidal thoughts and behavior
- Use liquid formulation for slow titration for ↑ or ↓
- Allow 2 to 4 weeks for full onset of therapeutic action
- Take with food if gastrointestinal upset
- If activating, recommend morning doses

PRESCRIBING FOR DEPRESSION

Tables 5.2 to 5.6 list antidepressant treatment options for children and adults with depression, dosage forms, recommended dosing and titration schedules, and maximum recommended dosages. Other medication classes can be used to treat and manage depression and are described in other chapters.

Serotonin-Norepinephrine Reuptake Inhibitors' Mechanism of Action

These inhibit the reabsorption of both serotonin and norepinephrine to the brain by blocking their reuptake pump or transport. Serotonin-norepinephrine reuptake inhibitors (SNRIs) depress the firing of serotonergic and norepinephrine neurons, desensitizing serotonin and norepinephrine receptors as a result.

Cautions to Take With Selective Serotonin Reuptake Inhibitors and Serotonin-Norepinephrine Reuptake Inhibitors

- Do not take SSRIs or SNRIs with monoamine oxidase inhibitors (MAOIs)
- Monitor blood pressure
- Assess for excessive alcohol use
- Assess risk of serotonin syndrome:
  - combined use of more than one SSRI
  - adjunct use of another antidepressant with SSRI
  - combining serotonergic drugs (i.e., combining St. John's wort, triptans, tricyclic antidepressants [TCAs], fentanyl, lithium, or tramadol with antidepressants)
- Discuss the risks of taking medicines during pregnancy
- Use with caution if you have narrow-angle glaucoma
- Note that SSRIs block serotonin reuptake in platelets and inhibit platelet aggregation; therefore, patients taking antiplatelet medications or patients with a personal history of inherited or acquired coagulopathies or platelet disorders, gastrointestinal bleeding, or intracranial hemorrhage should use caution when taking SSRIs.

Table 5.2

Selective Serotonin Reuptake Inhibitors (SSRIs)

Generic Name (Brand Name)	Dosage Forms	FDA Approval	Clinical Considerations
Citalopram (Celexa)	Tablet Solution	*Adults:* MDD *Non-FDA Uses:* alcoholism, OCD, panic disorders, PMDD, agitation from dementia, fibromyalgia *Off-Label:* alcoholism, binge-eating disorder, GAD, OCD, panic disorders, PMDD, hot flashes *Pediatrics:* safety in pediatric use has not been established *Off-Label:* MDD, impulsive aggressive behavior *Older Adult Considerations:* use lower doses of medication *,**,***	May take 4 to 6 weeks for full effect Monitor cardiac electrical activity dose-dependent prolongation of the corrected QT interval, which can lead to a life-threatening cardiac arrhythmia, torsade de pointes; observe/monitor for activation of suicidal ideation Observe/monitor for activation of bipolar disorder
Escitalopram (Lexapro)	Tablet Solution	*Adults:* MDD, GAD *Non-FDA Uses:* OCD, panic disorders, PMDD *Off-Label:* OCD, insomnia, vasomotor symptoms with menopause *Pediatrics:* MDD (≥12 years old) *Older Adult Considerations:* *,**,***	May take 2 to 4 weeks for full effect Instruct patient to take with food if GI upset Solution formulation for slow titration observe/monitor for activation of suicidal and bipolar disorder
Fluoxetine (Prozac)	Tablet Solution Capsule Capsule Weekly	*Adults:* MDD, bulimia nervosa, OCD, panic disorder, PMDD *Non-FDA Uses:* dysthymia, PTSD, fibromyalgia, body dysmorphic disorder, Raynaud phenomenon *Off-Label:* migraines, fibromyalgia, Raynaud phenomenon, hot flashes due to hormonal chemotherapy *Pediatrics:* MDD (≥8 years old), OCD (≥7 years old), body dysmorphic disorder *Older Adult Considerations:* *,**,***	First SSRI on the market Peak plasma levels in 6 to 8 hours Long half-life Considered "activating" compared to other SSRIs Solution formulation for slow titration Observe/monitor for activation of suicidal ideation bipolar disorder Observe/monitor for activation of bipolar disorder

*Start at lowest dosage and increase, if necessary, slowly while monitoring for side effects.
**May exacerbate or cause syndrome of inappropriate antidiuretic hormone secretion (SIADH) or hyponatremia in older adults; need to monitor sodium level closely when starting or changing dosages in older adults due to increased risk (Beers Criteria, 2012).
***Monitor renal and hepatic function; may require lower doses due to real and/or heaptatic impairments

(continued)

Table 5.2

Selective Serotonin Reuptake Inhibitors (SSRIs) (*continued*)

Generic Name (Brand Name)	Dosage Forms	FDA Approval	Clinical Considerations
Fluvoxamine (Luvox)	Tablet CR Capsule	*Adults:* OCD, social anxiety disorder *Non-FDA Uses:* panic disorder, eating disorders, PTSD *Pediatrics:* OCD (≥8 years) *Older Adult Considerations:* *,**,***	Can be given once a day or in divided doses Instruct patient to take at night to reduce side effects of drowsiness
Paroxetine (Paxil)	Suspension IR Tablet CR Tablet	*Adults:* MDD, GAD, OCD, panic disorder, PMDD, PTSD, social anxiety. *Non-FDA Uses:* premature ejaculation *Pediatrics:* safety in pediatric use has not been established *Off-Label:* stuttering, vasovagal syncope, diabetic neuropathy *Older Adult Considerations:* *,**,***	IR ties to paroxetine mesylate CR ties to paroxetine hydrochloride Contraindicated in pregnancy Taper off slowly to avoid side effects May cause sedation and anticholinergic effects
Sertraline (Zoloft)	Concentrate Tablet	*Adults:* MDD, OCD, panic disorder, premenstrual dysphoric disorder, PTSD, social anxiety *Non-FDA Uses:* dysthymia, GAD, night eating disorder *Off-Label:* pruritus *Pediatrics:* OCD (≥6 years) *Older Adult Considerations:* *,**,***	Instruct patient to take with food if GI upset If activating, advise patient to take in the morning

*Start at lowest dosage and increase, if necessary, slowly while monitoring for side effects.
**May exacerbate or cause syndrome of inappropriate antidiuretic hormone secretion (SIADH) or hyponatremia in older adults; need to monitor sodium level closely when starting or changing dosages in older adults due to increased risk (Beers Criteria, 2012).
***Monitor renal and hepatic function; may require lower doses due to real and/or heaptatic impairments.
CR, controlled release; FDA, U.S. Food and Drug Administration; GAD, general anxiety disorder; GI, gastrointestinal; IR, immediate release; MDD, major depressive disorder; OCD, obsessive-compulsive disorder; PMDD, premenstrual dysphoric disorder; PTSD, posttraumatic stress disorder.

TRICYCLIC ANTIDEPRESSANTS

Tricyclic antidepressants (TCAs) should be used with caution because of their potential side effects and risk profile. Some of the risks are associated with their ability to induce a blockade of α 1 adrenergic receptors (dizziness or hypotension), anticholinergic and sedating side effects, and narrow therapeutic index. Caution should be exercised with older adults in particular due to their increased risk of toxicity or death if TCA is taken in overdose to induce suicide. Providers should avoid prescribing TCAs to individuals with

Table 5.3

Serotonin and Norepinephrine Reuptake Inhibitors

Generic Name (Brand Name)	Dosage Forms	FDA Approval	Clinical Considerations
Desvenlafaxine (Pristiq, Khedezla)	Extended-Release Tablet	*Adults:* MDD *Non-FDA Uses:* premature ejaculation *Pediatrics:* safety in pediatric use has not been established *Older Adult Considerations:* *,**,***	Advise patient to swallow tablets whole without chewing, opening, or crushing Gradual taper is recommended when discontinuing
Duloxetine (Cymbalta, Drizalma Sprinkle)	Delayed Release Capsule	*Adults:* MDD, GAD, panic disorder, social anxiety disorder, fibromyalgia, diabetic neuropathy pain *Non-FDA Uses:* pain, urinary incontinence, premature ejaculation *Pediatrics:* safety in pediatric use has not been established GAD (≥7 years), fibromyalgia (≥13 years) *Older Adult Considerations:* *,**,***	Gradually taper when discontinuing
Levomilnacipran (Fetzima)	Extended-Release Capsule	*Adults:* MDD *Pediatrics:* safety in pediatric use has not been established *Older Adult Considerations:*	Swallow capsules – advise patients to not open, chew, or crush Gradual taper when discontinuing
Milnacipran (Savella)	Tablet	*Adults:* fibromyalgia *Pediatrics:* safety in pediatric use has not been established *Older Adult Considerations:* risk of hyponatremia, SIADH, or both may occur in older adult patients*,**,***	For older adults with renal impairment, lower divided doses

*Start at lowest dosage and increase, if necessary, slowly while monitoring for side effects.
**May exacerbate or cause syndrome of inappropriate antidiuretic hormone secretion (SIADH) or hyponatremia in older adults; need to monitor sodium level closely when starting or changing dosages in older adults due to increased risk (Beers Criteria, 2012).
***Monitor renal and hepatic function; may require lower doses due to real and/or heaptatic impairments.

(*continued*)

Table 5.3

Serotonin and Norepinephrine Reuptake Inhibitors (*continued*)

Generic Name (Brand Name)	Dosage Forms	FDA Approval	Clinical Considerations
Venlafaxine (Effexor)	Immediate Release Tablet Extended-Release Capsule Extended-Release Tablet	*Adults:* MDD, GAD, panic disorder, social anxiety disorder *Off-Label:* PTSD, neuropathic pain *Non-FDA Uses:* PTSD, OCD, ADHD, eating disorders, headaches, PMDD, premature ejaculation *Pediatrics:* safety in pediatric use has not been established *Off-Label:* ADD, anxiety disorders, depression *Older Adult Considerations:* *,**,***	Exhibits SSRI activity at lower doses (75 mg) and SNRI activity at moderate doses (150 to 225 mg) and inhibits dopamine reuptake at higher doses (375 mg) May result in a false positive for PCP in urine samples Taper slowly to avoid side effects

*Start at lowest dosage and increase, if necessary, slowly while monitoring for side effects.
**May exacerbate or cause syndrome of inappropriate antidiuretic hormone secretion (SIADH) or hyponatremia in older adults; need to monitor sodium level closely when starting or changing dosages in older adults due to increased risk (Beers Criteria, 2012).
***Monitor renal and hepatic function; may require lower doses due to real and/or heaptatic impairments.
ADD, attention deficit disorder; ADHD, attention deficit hyperactive disorder; FDA, U.S. Food and Drug Administration; GAD, general anxiety disorder; MDD, major depressive disorder; OCD, obsessive-compulsive disorder; PMDD, premenstrual dysphoric disorder; PTSD, posttraumatic stress disorder; SIADH, syndrome of inappropriate antidiuretic hormone; SNRI, serotonin and norepinephrine reuptake inhibitor; SSRI, selective serotonin reuptake inhibitor

cognitive impairment, cardiac conductive abnormalities, urinary retention, and chronic constipation. Additionally, TCAs may contribute to hypotension and therefore increase fall risk. Baseline EKG is recommended before the initiating TCAs. Table 5.4 lists TCAs and tetracyclic dosage information.

Tricyclic Mechanism of Action

Tricyclic drugs inhibit the cellular uptake and inactivation of serotonin and noradrenaline that contribute to elevated amounts of noradrenergic and serotonergic neurotransmission in the brain. Tricyclic drugs also work as an antagonist on postsynaptic alpha cholinergic muscarinic and histaminergic receptors.

Tricyclic Antidepressants Specific Adverse Effects

- Blurred vision
- Cardiovascular complications (arrhythmias, QTc prolongation, widened QRS complex, ventricular fibrillation, and sudden cardiac death in patients with preexisting heart disease)

Table 5.4

Tricyclic Antidepressants

Generic Name (Brand Name)	Dosage Forms	FDA Approval	Clinical Considerations
Amitriptyline (Elavil, Endep)	Tablet	*Adults:* MDD *Non-FDA Uses:* GAD, bulimia nervosa, PTSD, chronic pain, fibromyalgia, IBS *Off-Label:* post-herpetic neuralgia, migraine prophylaxis, eating disorders *Pediatrics:* safety in pediatric use under 12 years has not been established; MDD (over 12 years) *Off-Label:* MDD (children < 12 years), analgesia for chronic pain, migraine prophylaxis *Older Adult Considerations:* may be increased gradually *,**,***,****,*****	Assess cardiac function: cardiac arrhythmias (QT prolongation); drug interactions; older adults with risk of falls; and patients at high risk of overdose Inexpensive option as a sleep aid: low-dose amitriptyline typically 10–20 mg for insomnia
Clomipramine (Anafranil)	Capsule	*Adults:* OCD *Non-FDA Uses:* GAD, panic disorder, premenstrual dysphoric disorder, delusional disorder, depression, pervasive developmental disorder, chronic pain *Off-Label:* premature ejaculation *Pediatrics:* safety in pediatric use under 10 years has not been established; OCD (over 10 years) *Older Adult Considerations:* may be increased gradually*,**,***,****	Best to take at bedtime to avoid daytime drowsiness Monitor cardiac electrical activity
Desipramine (Norpramin)	Tablet	*Adults:* MDD *Non-FDA Uses:* GAD, bulimia nervosa, chronic pain, ADHD *Off-Label:* post-herpetic neuralgia, vulvodynia, eating disorders *Pediatrics:* safety in pediatric use under 12 years has not been established *Older Adult Considerations:* start with lowest dose* May be increased gradually*,**,***,****	Best to take at bedtime to avoid daytime drowsiness Monitor cardiac electrical activity Monitor for orthostatic hypotension

*Doses should be taken at bedtime due to sedative effects.
**Monitor renal and hepatic function; may require lower doses due to real and/or heaptatic impairments.
***Dose can be increased every 3 to 5 days while monitoring serum levels, efficacy, and side effects.
****Avoid in older adults with falls and/or fractures due to anticholinergic and sedative effects unless no other safer alternative is available (Beers Criteria, 2012).
*****TCA overdose can be fatal.

(*continued*)

Table 5.4

Tricyclic Antidepressants (*continued*)

Generic Name (Brand Name)	Dosage Forms	FDA Approval	Clinical Considerations
Imipramine (Tofranil)	Tablet Capsule	*Adults:* MDD, nocturnal enuresis *Non-FDA Uses:* GAD, bulimia nervosa, panic disorder, PTSD, social anxiety disorder, chronic pain, headache *Pediatrics:* safety in pediatric use under 12 years has not been established Nocturnal enuresis (over 6 years) *Off-Label:* depression, chronic pain *Older Adult Considerations:* start with lowest dose* May be increased gradually*,**,***,****	Best to take at bedtime to avoid daytime drowsiness Monitor cardiac electrical activity
Nortriptyline (Pamelor)	Capsule Oral Solution	*Adults:* MDD *Non-FDA Uses:* GAD, chronic pain, ADHD, nicotine dependence, nocturnal enuresis *Off-Label:* chronic urticaria, smoking cessation, ADHD, post-herpetic neuralgia *Pediatrics:* safety in pediatric use under 6 years has not been established. Over 12 years: 30 to 50 mg per day (divided)* *Off-Label:* depression, nocturnal enuresis, ADHD *Older Adult Considerations:* start with lowest dose.* May be increased gradually*,**,***,****	Best to take at bedtime to avoid daytime drowsiness Monitor cardiac electrical activity Monitor for orthostatic hypotension
Protriptyline (Vivactil)	Tablet: 5 mg 10 mg	*Adults:* MDD *Pediatrics:* safety in pediatric use under 12 years has not been established *FDA:* MDD (over 12 years); increase incrementally as tolerated** *Older Adult Considerations:* may be increased gradually*,**,***,****	Monitor cardiac electrical activity Monitor weight Less sedating than other TCAs
Trimipramine (Surmontil)	Capsule	*Adults:* MDD *Pediatrics:* safety in pediatric use under 12 years has not been established; MDD (over 12 years) increase incrementally as tolerated** *Older Adult Considerations:* may be increased gradually*,**,***,****	Best to take at bedtime to avoid daytime drowsiness May be given in divided doses Monitor cardiac electrical activity

*Doses should be taken at bedtime due to sedative effects.
**Start at lowest dosage and increase, if necessary, slowly while monitoring for side effects; can be increased every 3 to 5 days while monitoring serum levels, efficacy, and side effects.
***Avoid in older adults with falls and/or fractures due to anticholinergic and sedative effects unless no other safer alternative is available (Beers Criteria).
****TCA overdose can be fatal.
ADHD, attention deficit hyperactive disorder; FDA, U.S. Food and Drug Administration; GAD, general anxiety disorder; IBS, irritable bowel syndrome; MDD, major depressive disorder; OCD, obsessive-compulsive disorder; PTSD, post-traumatic stress disorder; TCA, tricyclic antidepressants

Table 5.5

Atypical Antidepressants and Noradrenergic and Specific Serotonergic Antidepressants

Generic Name (Brand Name)	Dosage Forms	FDA Approval	Nursing Considerations
Nefazodone (Serzone)	Tablet	*Adults:* MDD *Pediatrics:* safety in pediatric use has not been established *Older Adult Considerations:* *	Monitor for CNS, GI, and vision changes Can be administered with or without food
Trazodone (Desyrel)	IR Tablet XL Tablet	*Adults:* MDD *Non-FDA Uses:* insomnia *Off-Label:* insomnia, aggressive behavior, cocaine withdrawal, alcohol withdrawal, prevention of migraine *Pediatrics:* safety in pediatric use has not been established *Off-Label:* depression *Older Adult Considerations:* increased risk of side effects in older adults	Trazodone has similar properties to SSRIs with fewer side effects Increased risk of side effects in older adults
Vilazodone (Viibryd)	Tablet	*Adults:* MDD *Pediatrics:* safety in pediatric use has not been established *Older Adult Considerations:* *	Gradually taper Take with food
Vortioxetine (Brintellix)	Tablet	*Adults:* MDD *Pediatrics:* safety in pediatric use has not been established *Older Adult Considerations:* *	Long half-life of 66 hours
Mirtazapine (Remeron)	Tablet Disintegrating Tablet	*Adults:* MDD *Off-Label:* anxiety, OCD, panic disorder, PTSD, hot flashes, insomnia, sexual dysfunction *Pediatrics:* safety in pediatric use has not been established *Older Adult Considerations:* *	Monitor weight and lipid profile Medication usually given at night due to sedative effect Older adults may have increased plasma levels of the drug; stop MAOIs for 2 weeks before starting medication to avoid risk of serotinin syndrome

*Start at the lowest dosage and titrate slowly while monitoring the patient for any side effects. May have sedating effects.

(*continued*)

Table 5.5

Atypical Antidepressants and Noradrenergic and Specific Serotonergic Antidepressants (*continued*)

Generic Name (Brand Name)	Dosage Forms	FDA Approval	Nursing Considerations
Bupropion (Wellbutrin, Forfivo, Zyban, Aplenzin)	Wellbutrin IR Tablets SR Tablets XL Tablets Aplenzin Forfivo Zyban	*Adults:* MDD, seasonal affective disorder (extended-release formulations), smoking cessation (Zyban) *Non-FDA Uses:* ADHD, depression (with bipolar disorder), obesity, antidepressant-associated sexual dysfunction *Off-Label:* ADHD, neuropathic pain *Pediatrics:* safety in pediatric use has not been established *Off-Label:* ADHD	SL tablets should not exceed 200 mg in one dose XL tablets should not exceed 450 mg in one dose

*Start at the lowest dosage and titrate slowly while monitoring the patient for any side effects.
**Monitor for renal impairment
ADHD, attention deficit hyperactivity disorder; CNS, central nervous system; GI, gastrointestinal; FDA, U.S. Food and Drug Administration; IR, immediate release; MDD, major depressive disorder; OCD, obsessive-compulsive disorder; PTSD, posttraumatic stress disorder; SR, sustained release; SSRI, selective serotonin reuptake inhibitor; XL, extended release

- Confusion
- Constipation
- Dizziness
- Increased risk of seizures in those with epilepsy
- Myoclonus
- Orthostatic hypotension
- Sedation
- Tachycardia
- Urinary retention
- Weight gain
- Xerostomia

Essential Facts

Amoxapine should be avoided in patients who have Parkinson's disease due to its dopamine-receptor-blocking properties.

ATYPICAL ANTIPDEPRESSANTS

Vilazodone and Vortioxetine Mechanism of Action

Vilazodone is a combined serotonin 5-HT_{1A} auto-receptor partial agonist with serotonin reuptake inhibition (SPARI) properties, so it acts like an

Table 5.6

Monoamine Oxidase Inhibitors

Generic Name (Brand Name)	Dosage Forms	FDA Approval	Nursing Considerations
Isocarboxazid (Marplan)	Tablet	*Adults:* depression *Pediatrics:* safety in pediatric use has not been established; depression (16 years and older) *Older Adult Considerations:* *	Monitor BP for orthostatic hypotension, sedation, weight gain
Phenelzine (Nardil)	Tablet	*Adults:* depression *Non-FDA Use:* anxiety disorders, bulimia nervosa, PTSD *Pediatrics:* safety in pediatric use has not been established *Older Adult Considerations:* *	Monitor BP for orthostatic hypotension, sedation, weight gain
Selegiline (Emsam)	Tablet/ Capsule Patch	*Adults:* depression, Parkinson's disease (oral) *Non-FDA Use:* Alzheimer disease *Pediatrics:* safety in pediatric use has not been established *Older Adult Considerations:* *	May result in a false positive for amphetamines/ methamphetamines in urine samples
Tranylcypromine (Parnate)	Tablet	*Adults:* depression *Pediatrics:* safety in pediatric use has not been established *Older Adult Considerations:* *	Monitor BP for orthostatic hypotension, sedation, weight gain

*Start with lowest possible dose and increase gradually while monitoring side effects, which may include orthostatic hypotension and potential drug–drug interactions

Note: Monoamine oxidase inhibitors should be used in patients who have had unsatisfactory results from other antidepressants.

BP, blood pressure; FDA, U.S. Food and Drug Administration; PTSD, posttraumatic stress disorder

SSRI but also has direct serotonin receptor interactions. Vilazodone boosts serotonin release within the brain's serotonergic pathways by blocking serotonin transporters, and simultaneously stimulates serotonin-1a receptors via partial agonism (Schwartz et al., 2011). The dosage information for vilazodone can be found in Table 5.5.

Vortioxetine, serotonin modulator and stimulator, has a unique pharmacologic profile, and its mechanism of action is not fully understood. Vortioxetine's antidepressant action is thought to be associated with its direct modulation of serotonergic receptor (5-HT) activity and serotonin transporter (SERT) inhibition along with its serotonin (5-HT) receptor agonism (5-HT1A), which boosts downregulation of presynaptic 5-HT1A receptors to disinhibit serotonin release; serotonin (5-HT) receptor *partial* agonism (5-HT1B), adding to its antidepressant properties; serotonin (5-HT) receptor antagonism (5-HT3), which theoretically reduces nausea and vomiting (nausea and vomiting can be unwanted side effects from ingesting vortioxetine); 5-HT1D antagonism, playing a role in anxiety levels and leading to vascular vasoconstriction in the brain; and 5-HT7 antagonism, which, although not clinically proven, hypothetically provides procognitive effects (Koesters et al., 2017). The dosage information for vortioxetine can be found in Table 5.5.

Nefazodone Mechanism of Action

Nefazodone is an atypical antidepressant that inhibits the reuptake of serotonin and norepinephrine by antagonizing the postsynaptic 5-HT_2 receptor and α_1-adrenergic receptors. Since nefazodone inhibits cytochrome P450, caution should be used when nefazodone is used together with other medications metabolized by the cytochrome P450 isoenzyme to avoid potential adverse interactions. Additionally, individuals with liver function impairments should avoid using nefazodone. Drugs to avoid with use of nefazodone include reductase inhibitors, carbamazepine, and macrolide antibiotics. The dosage information for nefazodone is provided in Table 5.5.

Trazodone Mechanism of Action

Trazodone's blockade of serotonin 5-HT2A receptors is its main function; however, its mechanism of action is not fully understood. At lower doses (25–100 mg), 5-HT2A, histamine H1, and alpha receptors produce the hypnotic effects. Blocking of 5-HT2A and serotonin reuptake transport occurs with higher doses in the 150 mg to 600 mg range (Jaffer et al., 2017). The dosage information for trazodone can be found in Table 5.5.

- Antagonist at the serotonin type 2 (5-HT2) receptors
- Antagonist at the alpha1 (α1) adrenergic receptors
- Inhibitors of serotonin reuptake transporter
- Moderator of cortisol suppression
- Modest antihistamine activity
- Low anticholinergic activity
- Hypnotic effect and antidepressant effects

Essential Facts

Trazodone has a mild side-effect profile, with sedation as the most common side effect.

Mirtazapine Mechanism of Action

Mirtazapine is a noradrenergic and specific serotonergic antidepressant that has a small effect on monoamine reuptake and produces antagonism of (a) central α 2-adrenergic auto-receptors, (b) heteroreceptors, (c) serotonin 5-hydroxytryptamine-2 (5-HT2), and (d) 5-HT3 receptors (Watanabe et al., 2011). Antagonism of α 2-adrenergic receptors results in a blockade of presynaptic autoreceptors, boosts norepinephrine release, and blocks heteroreceptors on serotonin neurons, which increases serotonin release (Watanabe et al., 2011). Potential side effects include dry mouth, sedation, increases in appetite, weight gain, sexual side effects, drowsiness, fall risk in older adults, fatigue, hypotension, constipation, and dry mouth. The dosage information for mirtazapine can be found in Table 5.5.

Essential Facts

Lower doses of mirtazapine induce antihistaminergic effects, causing sleepiness and drowsiness; however, higher doses produce more noradrenergic neurotransmission that counteracts some of the antihistaminergic properties.

Norepinephrine Dopamine Reuptake Inhibitor Mechanism of Action

Bupropion enhances monoaminergic neurotransmission via its effects on norepinephrine (NE) and dopamine (DA) by presynaptic reuptake inhibition. With similar efficacy to SSRIs in the treatment for depression, bupropion is the only antidepressant with negligible effects on serotonin, histamine, acetylcholine, or adrenaline (epinephrine) neurotransmission; therefore, bupropion is less sedating than SSRIs and other antidepressants (Patel et al., 2016). Generally, bupropion is well tolerated in short- and longer-term administration. Other uses for bupropion include adjunctive treatment to reverse antidepressant-induced sexual dysfunction and to augment antidepressant efficacy. Bupropion side effects include headache, elevated blood pressure, dry mouth, nausea, insomnia, constipation, dizziness, seizure (rare), tachycardia/dysrhythmia, weight loss, tinnitus, anxiety, and agitation. The dosage information for bupropion can be found in Table 5.5.

Essential Facts

Compared to other antidepressants, bupropion has low incidence of the following:

- Sexual dysfunction
- Weight gain
- Drowsiness

Monoamine Oxidase Inhibitors (MAOIs) Mechanism of Action

The monoamine theory of depression suggests that monoamine levels (noradrenaline, dopamine, and serotonin) are lowered in depression. Notably, there are two monoamine oxidase (MAO) enzyme isomers: MAO-A and MAO-B. MAO-A is found in the gut, liver, placenta, and the parts of the brain that have serotonin, norepinephrine, dopamine, and tyramine substrates. MAO-B is primarily found in platelets, the liver, and in dense dopaminergic regions of the brain and results in antiparkinsonian activity. Furthermore, MAOIs influence noradrenaline, dopamine, and serotonin—the neurotransmitters associated with depression—by blocking monoamine oxidase enzyme and increasing synaptic availability.

MAOIs have been shown to be effective in treating depression; however, due to the large number of potential interactions between prescription and nonprescription medications and dietary interactions, they are prescribed with caution. Due to drug and food interactions, MAOIs are typically not firstline agents and are generally restricted for (a) individuals who experienced numerous unsuccessful trials of antidepressants or (b) individuals who present with atypical depressive symptoms (Ramsay & Tipton, 2017). When MAO enzymes are inhibited and tyramine (a precursor to norepinephrine) is ingested, tyramine levels rise and employ a robust vasopressor response that leads to elevated levels of circulating catecholamines (epinephrine and norepinephrine), leading to abrupt heart-rate escalation and elevated blood pressure. Nurse practitioners must provide education about MAOIs to patients and caregivers, discuss the associated risks, and monitor for adverse effects. Tyramine can increase with the aging of food; thus, individuals should be encouraged to eat fresh foods. The dosage information for MAOIs can be found in Table 5.6.

Essential Facts

The primary diagnosis of MDD should be confirmed in individuals who exhibit treatment-resistant depression.

Monoamine Oxidase Inhibitors Diet and Medications Restrictions

A tyramine content of less than 6 mg per serving is generally considered safe. The following sections detail the foods and medications to avoid when taking MAOIs and the possible side effects of MAOIs.

Tyramine-Free Diet: Foods to Avoid

- Aged wine and other alcoholic beverages
- Aged cheese (smoked, processed, marinated)
- Fava beans
- Meats and fish (smoked, processed, marinated, sausage, turkey, liver, and salami)
- Overripe fruits (apricots, raisins, figs, bananas)
- Tap beer (contains tyramine)
- Sauerkraut

Medications to Avoid When Taking Monoamine Oxidase Inhibitors

- SSRIs
- SNRIs
- TCAs

- Bupropion
- Mirtazapine
- St. John's wort
- Dextromethorphan (over-the-counter [OTC] cold and allergy medications)
- Tramadol
- Meperidine
- Methadone
- Stimulants
- Adrenergic and serotonergic medications

Monoamine Oxidase Inhibitor Side Effects

- Agitation
- Flushing
- Heightened deep tendon reflexes
- High fevers
- Hypertensive crisis
- Hypotension or hypertension
- Muscle pain
- Nausea
- Palpations
- Seizures
- Serotonin syndrome
- Sexual dysfunction
- Tachycardia
- Twitching
- Weight gain
- May be lethal in overdose
- Effects can take 2 to 3 weeks; more than 6 months for maximum effects with an increased risk of relapse if taken for fewer than 6 months

Essential Facts

Combining serotonergic antidepressants and other serotonergic medications with MAOIs involves the risk of serotonin syndrome.

Although antidepressants have been shown to be effective in the treatment of depression, like all medications they can produce mild to severe unwanted or bothersome adverse effects. Generally, mild side effects dissipate or become less severe over time.

General Antidepressant Side Effects

- Activation of mania
- Agitation/anxiety
- Arrhythmias, QT prolongation
- Blood pressure changes (orthostatic hypotension)

- Falls/fractures
- Fatigue
- GI distress or nausea
- Headache
- Hyponatremia/syndrome of inappropriate antidiuretic hormone secretion (SIADH)
- Insomnia
- Nervousness or jitteriness
- Sexual dysfunction (dysorgasmia, loss of libido, impotence)
- Sweating
- Suicide/suicidal ideation/suicide attempts
- Tremor (shaking)
- Weight loss or gain

Less Common, but Serious, Side Effects of Antidepressant Use

- Abnormal bleeding or bruising
- Akathisia (cannot sit still)
- Seizures
- Serotonin syndrome
- Tinnitus
- Withdrawal symptoms

Essential Facts

Depression is the most common psychiatric disorder in older adults and occurs more often than dementia. Associated factors in older adults with depression include the following:

- Chronic health problems
- Cognitive impairments
- Functional impairment
- Lack of close social contacts
- More prone to cardiovascular events and have a higher risk of anticholinergic and cognitive decline related to antidepressant use
- Personal history of depression

Together, clinicians and patients must carefully weigh both the benefits and potential harms.

THE WASHOUT PERIOD

A *washout period* is a predefined period of time before or during treatment when individuals receive no active medication. In psychiatry, the washout period is used to distinguish medication effects and their adverse reactions from psychiatric symptoms. Washout periods are useful in children or adolescents before their brains have matured, in individuals using street drugs, or in individuals in the midst of a hormonal storm. Comparative estimates of washout-period intolerance are 5.9% to 7.8% compared to estimates of polypharmacy intolerance of 9.1% to 34.1% (Hoffman et al., 2011). The following are the risks to washing out medications:

- Discontinuation symptoms
- Fears
- Inpatient versus outpatient status
- Relapse
- Return or rebound of their medical/psychiatric problems
- Severity of illness and/or speed of withdrawal
- Withdrawal (particularly with benzodiazepines)
- Withdrawal symptoms

Required Washout Times Between Changes in Antidepressant Prescribing

- At minimum, five half-lives should elapse between stopping an SSRI and starting MAOI
- Drugs with long half-life metabolites → MAOI (example: fluoxetine)
  - 5- to 6-week washout period
- Drugs with short half-life metabolites → MAOI (Example: venlafaxine, TCAs, etc.)
  - 2-week washout period
- MAOI → another MAOI
  - 2-week washout period
- MAOI → non-MAOI (SSRI)
  - 2-week washout period

Essential Facts

Polypharmacy is characterized as the concurrent use of multiple medications in a single patient, or combining of medications to enhance a response or cause the remission of psychiatric symptoms.

PRINCIPLES OF RATIONAL AND IRRATIONAL POLYPHARMACY

Depending on the situation, the term *polypharmacy* has evolved to characterize (a) simultaneous use of five or more medications, (b) multiple-drug consumption, (c) excessive use of drugs, (d) unnecessary drug use, or (e) the prescribing of medication without an indication (Varghese et al., 2021). Concurrent use of multiple medications increases the potential for higher rates of drug–drug interactions, nonadherence, and poorer health outcomes. According to Varghese et al. (2021) and Masnoon et al. (2017), in older adults, polypharmacy is associated with increases in reported falls, frailty, disability, increased length of stay in hospital and readmission to hospital soon after discharge, and mortality. *Rational polypharmacy* is guided by a set of prescribing principles that are considered when adding new medications. These principles include the use of (a) data from clinical trials and evidence of effectiveness, (b) knowledge of pharmacodynamic and/or pharmacokinetic drug interactions, (c) risk versus safety profile, (d) potential drug interactions, (e) cost-effectiveness, and (f) shared decision-making. *Irrational polypharmacy* refers to the practice of prescribing multiple medications due to (a) lack of understanding of pharmacology and risk-to-benefit ratio, (b) apprehension or fear of changing or eliminating one of the medications, or (c) laziness.

KEY PRINCIPLES FOR MONITORING THERAPEUTIC RESPONSE

Patients should be monitored more frequently immediately after an acute phase of treatment, at the start of medication treatment, or after changes in treatment and characteristics of the individual patient. It is important to systematically monitor for treatment response or effectiveness, side effects, self-harm, suicidality, and other safety concerns on a regular basis (Kennedy et al., 2016; Sobieraj et al., 2009). In depressed individuals, medication titration to a full therapeutic dose is dependent upon age treatment setting, side effect risk profile, presence of co-occurring medical conditions, and pharmacotherapy. Other considerations for evaluation include available support, compliance and cooperation with treatment, and severity of the side effect risk profile.

To reduce the risk of relapse after remission, individuals who have been treated successfully with antidepressant medications during the acute phase of depression should continue medication treatment based on personal risk factors (Lam et al., 2016; Severe et al., 2020). Risk factors for chronic depression or relapses include childhood or adolescent onset, frequency and severity of depressive occurrences, sleep cycle disturbance, comorbid mental or physical illnesses, family history, social support, and stressful life events (Lam et al., 2016; Severe et al., 2020).

Essential Facts

The goal of antidepressant therapy is complete remission of symptoms and restoration of normal personal, social, and occupational functioning. Individuals who experience a 50% or more reduction in baseline symptom levels are categorized as having a significant response to treatment (O'Connor et al., 2009).

Ongoing medication therapy is recommended for individuals who (a) are diagnosed with MDD, (b) have experienced three or more major depressive episodes, (c) have ongoing psychologic stressors, and (d) have a family history of depression. In addition, the different levels of care and optimal treatment settings for each individual should be reevaluated on an ongoing basis throughout the course of treatment. Furthermore, to enable clinicians to make informed decisions throughout the treatment process, continuous systematic monitoring of patient outcomes includes (a) utilizing measurement-based tools or validated rating scale, (b) tracking of depressive symptoms, (c) monitoring side effects, (d) assessment of treatment adherence, (e) ongoing evaluation of self-harm and suicide risk (suicidal thoughts, intent, plans, means, and behaviors), (f) clinical decision-making based on response to therapeutic goals, (g) ongoing patient and caregiver education; and (h) involvement of patients and/or caregivers in decision-making processes (Lam et al., 2016; Parikh et al., 2009; Severe et al., 2020; Sobieraj et al., 2009).

For Optimal Patient Outcomes, Ongoing Monitoring for Patient Management Also Includes:

- Assessment of past and recent suicidal behavior (family history of suicide)
- Assessment of patient safety
- Assessment of treatment barriers (economic, cultural, logistical, motivational, etc.)
- Continued monitoring of co-occurring psychiatric and/or medical conditions, work, school, family, social relationships, and leisure activities
- Delineation of current stressors
- Risk of harm to oneself or others
- Identification of specific psychiatric symptoms (e.g., psychosis, severe anxiety, substance use)
- Maintenance of health and hygiene; assess level of self-care, hydration, and nutrition
- Protective factors such as positive reasons for living, as well as strong familial and/or social support

The decision as to when to terminate antidepressant treatment is patient-centric; therefore, for optimal outcomes the decision is based on the patient's risk of recurrence, history of recurrent depression, concurrent psychiatric illness (anxiety), type of depression of symptoms, family and social support, and presence of other medical illnesses that indicate an increased likelihood of relapse (Lam et al., 2016; Parikh et al., 2009).

GENERAL PRINCIPLES TO TERMINATE ANTIDEPRESSANT TREATMENT DUE TO ACHIEVED RESPONSE

- Adherence to psychotherapy sessions
- Consider tapered withdrawal to prevent an unpleasant discontinuation syndrome
- Development of adverse consequences that interfere with treatments used for other medical conditions
- Drug–drug interactions
- Low profile of risk factors for recurrent MDD
- Persistent and intolerable side effects
- Reasonably justified by patient's strongly stated preference

INDICATIONS FOR REFERRALS

Although depression is generally treated on an outpatient basis, there are instances when hospitalization is necessary. When considering hospitalization, the single most important determinant is the patient's risk of self-harm or threat to harm oneself or others. Other considerations include new-onset psychosis, multiple treatment attempt failures, lack of adequate response to outpatient treatment, and lack of adequate support.

SUMMARY

Depression is a persistent disease that places a heavy burden on both individuals and society. Early recognition and early adequate treatment strategies at illness onset have been shown to improve outcomes. A large number of different interventions exist for the treatment of unipolar depression, including psychologic and pharmacologic therapies. Although the exact therapeutic mechanisms of antidepressants are not yet clear, it is clear that antidepressants have mood-enhancing, anxiolytic, or calming properties. The ultimate goal of treatment is safety, to diminish depressive symptomology, restore psychosocial functioning, and prevent reoccurrence (Machmutow et al., 2019).

RESOURCES

- National Pregnancy Registry for Antidepressants: 1-844-405-6185
- Substance Abuse and Mental Health Services Administration's (SAMHSA) National Helpline: 1-800-662-HELP (4357)
- Treatment Referral Routing Service : 1-800-487-4889 (service in English and Spanish)
- Mental Health America mental health support and discussion community: www.inspire.com/groups/mental-health-america/topic/depression/?origin=tfr
- National Institute of Mental Health: www.nimh.nih.gov/index.shtml

REVIEW QUESTIONS

1. Which one of the following statements about tricyclic antidepressants is true?
    a. Tricyclic antidepressants are to be used with caution due to inducing a blockade of α1 adrenergic receptors (dizziness or hypotension), their anticholinergic and sedating side effects, and narrow therapeutic index.
    b. Tricyclic antidepressants are generally safe in overdose.
    c. Tricyclic antidepressants are less sedating than SSRIs and other antidepressants.
    d. Tricyclic antidepressants are safe in older adults with depression.
2. Which one of the following statements regarding antidepressants is false?
    a. SSRIs are often firstline medication treatment for depression.

b. The exact therapeutic mechanisms of antidepressants are not yet clear, but they have mood-enhancing, anxiolytic, or calming properties.
c. There are three SSRIs that are FDA approved for children: fluoxetine, escitalopram, and bupropion.
d. Fluoxetine has a longer half-life than other SSRIs.

3. Decisions to terminate treatment for a 25-year-old female, who attends her appointments with her mother, should be based on which one of the following?
   a. Risk of recurrence and persistent symptoms
   b. Risk of recurrence and history of payment
   c. Mother's preference only
   d. Risk of recurrence, persistent symptoms, and mother's preference
4. A 34-year-old male reports that he feels "tired, sluggish, lacks motivation and has gained 8 pounds over the past few months." He also reports that he has not had a physical exam in over 2 years but thinks he has depression. Which one of the following laboratory test results should be checked before initiating antidepressant medications? Choose the best answer.
   a. Urinalysis and urine culture
   b. Vitamin D level
   c. Thyroid-stimulating hormone
   d. None are needed, just start a SSRI
5. When considering a SSRI for a 17-year-old male with depression who sometimes forgets to take his medication, which one of the following SSRIs would be considered due to its long half-life?
   a. Duloxetine
   b. Sertraline
   c. Fluoxetine
   d. Bupropion

REFERENCES

American Psychiatric Association. (2013). *Diagnostic and statistical manual of mental disorders* (5th ed.). https://doi.org/10.1176/appi.books.9780890425596

American Geriatrics Society Beers Criteria® Update Expert Panel (2019). American Geriatrics Society 2019 Updated AGS Beers Criteria® for Potentially Inappropriate Medication Use in Older Adults. *Journal of the American Geriatrics Society, 67*(4), 674–694. https://doi.org/10.1111/jgs.15767

Gautam, S., Jain, A., Gautam, M., Vahia, V. N., & Grover, S. (2017). Clinical practice guidelines for the management of depression. *Indian Journal of Psychiatry, 59*(Suppl. 1), S34–S50. https://doi.org/10.4103/0019-5545.196973

Hoffman, D. A., Schiller, M., Greenblatt, J. M., & Iosifescu, D. V. (2011). Polypharmacy or medication washout: An old tool revisited. *Neuropsychiatric Disease and Treatment, 7*(1), 639–648. https://doi.org/10.2147/NDT.S24375

Jaffer, K. Y., Chang, T., Vanle, B., Dang, J., Steiner, A. J., Loera, N., Abdelmesseh, M., Danovitch, I., & Ishak, W. W. (2017). Trazodone for insomnia: A systematic review. *Innovations in Clinical Neuroscience, 14*(7–8), 24–34. https://www.ncbi.nlm.nih.gov/pmc/articles/PMC5842888

Kennedy, S. H., Lam, R. W., McIntyre, R. S., Tourjman, S. V., Bhat, V., Blier, P., Hasnain, M., Jollant, F., Levitt, A. J., MacQueen, G. M., McInerney, S. J.,

McIntosh, D., Milev, R. V., Müller, D. J., Parikh, S. V., Pearson, N. L., Ravindran, A. V., Uher, R., & CANMAT Depression Work Group. (2016). Canadian Network for Mood and Anxiety Treatments (CANMAT) 2016 clinical guidelines for the management of adults with major depressive disorder: Section 3. Pharmacological treatments. *Canadian Journal of Psychiatry*, *61*(9), 540–560. https://doi.org/10.1177/0706743716659417

Koesters, M., Ostuzzi, G., Guaiana, G., Breilmann, J., & Barbui, C. (2017). Vortioxetine for depression in adults. *Cochrane Database of Systematic Reviews*, *7*(7), Article CD011520. https://doi.org/10.1002/14651858.CD011520.pub2

Lam, R. W., McIntosh, D., Wang, J., Enns, M. W., Kolivakis, T., Michalak, E. E., Sareen, J., Song, W. Y., Kennedy, S. H., MacQueen, G. M., Milev, R. V., Parikh, S. V., Ravindran, A. V., & CANMAT Depression Work Group. (2016). Canadian Network for Mood and Anxiety Treatments (CANMAT) 2016 clinical guidelines for the management of adults with major depressive disorder: Section 1. Disease burden and principles of care. *Canadian Journal of Psychiatry*, *61*(9), 510–523. https://doi.org/10.1177/0706743716659416

Machmutow, K., Meister, R., Jansen, A., Kriston, L., Watzke, B., Härter, M. C., & Liebherz, S. (2019). Comparative effectiveness of continuation and maintenance treatments for persistent depressive disorder in adults. *Cochrane Database of Systematic Reviews*, *5*(5), Article CD012855. https://doi.org/10.1002/14651858.CD012855.pub2

Masnoon, N., Shakib, S., Kalisch-Ellett, L., & Caughey, G. E. (2017). What is polypharmacy? A systematic review of definitions. *BMC Geriatrics*, *17*(1), 230. https://doi.org/10.1186/s12877-017-0621-2

Mullen, S. (2018). Major depressive disorder in children and adolescents. *Mental Health Clinician*, *8*(6), 275–283. https://doi.org/10.9740/mhc.2018.11.275

O'Connor, E. A., Whitlock, E. P., Gaynes, B., & Bell, T. L. (2009). *Screening for depression in adults and older adults in primary care: An updated systematic review* (Report No. 10-05143-EF-1). Agency for Healthcare Research and Quality.

Parikh, S. V., Segal, Z. V., Grigoriadis, S., Ravindran, A. V., Kennedy, S. H., Lam, R. W., Patten, S. B. (2009). Canadian Network for Mood and Anxiety Treatments (CANMAT) clinical guidelines for the management of major depressive disorder in adults. II. Psychotherapy alone or in combination with antidepressant medication. *Journal of Affective Disorders*, *117*(Suppl. 1), S15–S25. https://doi.org/10.1016/j.jad.2009.06.042

Patel, K., Allen, S., Haque, M. N., Angelescu, I., Baumeister, D., & Tracy, D. K. (2016). Bupropion: A systematic review and meta-analysis of effectiveness as an antidepressant. *Therapeutic Advances in Psychopharmacology*, *6*(2), 99–144. https://doi.org/10.1177/2045125316629071

Ramsay, R. R., & Tipton, K. F. (2017). Assessment of enzyme inhibition: A review with examples from the development of monoamine oxidase and cholinesterase inhibitory drugs. *Molecules*, *22*(7), Article 1192. https://doi.org/10.3390/molecules22071192

Schwartz, T. L., Siddiqui, U. A., & Stahl, S. M. (2011). Vilazodone: A brief pharmacological and clinical review of the novel serotonin partial agonist and reuptake inhibitor. *Therapeutic Advances in Psychopharmacology*, *1*(3), 81–87. https://doi.org/10.1177/2045125311409486

Severe, J., Greden, J. F., & Reddy, P. (2020). Consequences of recurrence of major depressive disorder: Is stopping effective antidepressant medications ever safe? *Focus*, *18*(2), 120–128. https://doi.org/10.1176/appi.focus.20200008

Sobieraj, D. M., Martinez, B. K., Hernandez, A. V., Coleman, C. I., Ross, J. S., Berg, K. M., Steffens, D. C., & Baker, W. L. (2009). Adverse effects of pharmacologic treatments of major depression in older adults. *Journal of the American Geriatric Society, 67*(8), 1571–1581. https://doi.org/10.1111/jgs.15966

Varghese, D., Ishida, C., & Haseer Koya, H. (2021). Polypharmacy. In: *StatPearls [Internet]*. StatPearls Publishing. https://www.ncbi.nlm.nih.gov/books/NBK532953

Watanabe, N., Omori, I. M., Nakagawa, A., Cipriani, A., Barbui, C., Churchill, R., & Furukawa, T. A. (2011). Mirtazapine versus other antidepressive agents for depression. *Cochrane Database of Systematic Reviews, 12*, Article CD006528. https://doi.org/10.1002/14651858.CD006528.pub2

6

Anxiolytics and Anti-Anxiety Medications

Anxiety disorders, which can range from mild to severe, impact both children and adults and are among the most prevalent mental health disorders worldwide. Anxiety disorders that manifest in childhood are linked with educational underachievement, co-occurring psychiatric conditions, significant functional impairment, increased risk for substance misuse, and negative outcomes later in life (Katzman et al., 2014; Reardon et al., 2019). Anxiety encompasses a heterogeneous group of conditions that can be characterized by a state of pervasive, unwarranted worry, nervousness, apprehension, and uneasiness that is difficult to control, causes significant distress and impairment, and occurs on more days than not over a period of 6 months. Acute attacks of anxiety include periods of intense motor and visceral activation, distortions of perception, loss of concentration, and impaired cognition, and may result in temporary debilitation (Kuang et al., 2017). Risk factors that place younger individuals at risk for anxiety include biologic influences, temperament, and environmental factors, such as stressful life experiences, parenting behaviors, and modeling.

In this chapter you will learn:

1. How to compare pharmacologic options for anxiety
2. How to name five or more criteria for generalized anxiety disorder
3. How to identify screening tools for anxiety-related disorders
4. How to evaluate medication safety considerations in anxiety management
5. How to assess therapeutic responses in anxious individuals

Anxious individuals have recurrent thoughts and catastrophic thinking patterns that focus on impending threats. Anxious individuals also engage in avoidant behaviors or behavioral adaptations and may complain of fatigue, muscle tension, or other somatic concerns. Similar to depression, monoaminergic systems play a major role in anxiety-related disorders (see Tables 6.1 to 6.3). The neurotransmitters primarily associated with anxiety-related disorders include gamma-aminobutyric acid (GABA), serotonin (5-HTP), norepinephrine (NE), and dopamine (DA). Abnormalities in the glutamate system are inherent to the pathophysiology of anxiety and other anxiety-related disorders. Generalized anxiety disorder (GAD) is the most common anxiety disorder, followed by phobias, panic disorder, and obsessive-compulsive disorders (OCD; Subramanyam et al., 2018). This chapter will cover psychotropic medications for use with GAD and other anxiety-related disorders, including OCD and posttraumatic stress disorder (PTSD).

DIAGNOSTIC CRITERIA FOR ANXIETY-RELATED DISORDERS

According to the *Diagnostic and Statistical Manual of Mental Disorders* (5th ed.; *DSM-5*; American Psychiatric Association [APA], 2013), the criterion for GAD is a pattern of difficult to control, frequent, excessive, and persistent worry that occurs more days than not for at least 6 months throughout activities or engagements. Worry due to GAD is not due to substance misuse, medication, or another medical or mental condition. This intense worry or

Table 6.1

Anxiety-Related Disorders

Disorder	Key Features
Separation anxiety disorder	Recurrent excessive distress (beyond clingy or easily homesick) when anticipating or experiencing separation from home, parent, or other major attachment figures
Selective mutism	Persistent failure to speak in select social settings despite having the ability to speak in more familiar settings
Specific phobia	Irrational or extreme fearful reactions to an object or situation (animals, heights, flying, seeing needles)
Social anxiety disorder (social phobia)	Intense fear or worry about personal functioning in social interactions (i.e., exceedingly self-conscious and afraid of being humiliated or doing something embarrassing)
Panic disorder	Recurrent and unexpected panic episodes (brief with rapid onset and include symptoms such as racing heart, chest pain, sweating, shaking, etc.) along with periods of intense worry about future attacks or fear of loss of control, resulting in avoidance behaviors
Agoraphobia	Marked fear and anxiety from being in places or situations where it is difficult to seek help if panic-like symptoms occur

Table 6.2

Obsessive-Compulsive-Related Disorders

Disorder	Key Features
Obsessive-compulsive disorder	The core symptoms include uncontrollable obsessions (compulsions; intrusive repetitive thoughts, urges, images; or impulses that trigger anxiety) and compulsions (repetitive behaviors or mental acts) that occur in response to obsessions
Body dysmorphic disorder	Preoccupation with actual or perceived flaws in physical appearance
Hoarding disorder	The accumulation of possessions hinders living functions as a result of having difficulty discarding possessions
Excoriation (skin-picking disorder)	Functional impairment and/or distress due to repetitive picking of one's skin
Trichotillomania (hair-pulling disorder)	Failure to resist urges to pull out one's own hair, leading to functional impairment and/or distress
Substance/medication-induced obsessive-compulsive disorder (OCRD) and related disorders	Onset of symptoms is induced by the consumption, inhalation, or injection of a substance

Table 6.3

Trauma- and Stressor-Related Disorders

Disorder	Key Features
Posttraumatic stress disorder	Develops following the exposure to severe trauma and is associated with intrusive memories, distressing dreams, dissociative reactions, avoidance of trauma-related stimuli, and increased arousal and irritability that negatively impact functioning
Disinhibited social engagement disorder	Socially atypical behaviors such as wandering away from a caregiver, readiness to depart with strangers, and engagement in overly familiar physical behaviors such as hugging or close physical contact with unfamiliar adults
Reactive attachment disorder	Emotionally withdrawn behaviors toward adult caregivers, persistent social or emotional disturbances, and display of minimal social and emotional openness and limited positive affect
Acute stress disorder	Symptomatology appears within 1 hour of the occurrence of a severe stress or traumatic event (e.g., natural disaster, accident) with symptoms beginning to subside within 48 hours
Adjustment disorders	Subsequent to a major psychosocial stressor or life event (e.g., divorce, illness), symptoms present with onset within 1 month of the major life event and generally subside by 6 months

apprehension causes significant impairment in personal, social, and occupational functioning and is associated with at least one of the following symptoms in children and at least three of the following symptoms in adults.

- Easily tired, worn-out, or fatigued
- Irritability
- Muscle tension
- Restlessness, uneasiness, or feeling on edge
- Sleep disturbance
- Struggle with concentrating or memory

Essential Facts

In order to differentiate everyday mild anxiety from pathologic anxiety, assess for significant distress or impairment in social, occupational, and overall personal functioning.

Other anxiety-related disorders include substance/medication-induced anxiety disorder, anxiety disorder due to another medical condition, other specified anxiety disorder, and unspecified anxiety disorder. The criteria for OCD, PTSD, and related trauma- and stressor-related disorders are in separate chapters of the *DSM-5*.

DIAGNOSTIC CRITERIA FOR OBSESSIVE-COMPULSIVE-RELATED DISORDERS

Other obsessive-compulsive-related disorders include obsessive-compulsive-related disorder due to another medical condition, other specified obsessive-compulsive-related disorder unspecified, and obsessive-compulsive-related disorder.

Essential Facts

In OCD, intrusive thoughts and repetitive behaviors are time consuming (e.g., more than an hour per day), distressing, or cause significant interference in functioning.

DIAGNOSTIC CRITERIA FOR TRAUMA- AND STRESSOR-RELATED DISORDERS

Other trauma- and stressor-related disorders include other specified trauma- and stressor-related disorder and unspecified trauma- and stressor-related disorder.

SCREENING TOOLS

- There are no laboratory tests specific to anxiety.
- Perform a baseline screening with a tool and repeat throughout the course of treatment to evaluate initial symptoms and response to treatment.

Pediatric Screening Tools

- Anxiety Disorders Interview Schedule Child and Parent Interviews (ADIS-C/P)
- Generalized Anxiety Disorder-7 (GAD-7)
- Hamilton Anxiety Scale (HAM-A)
- Preschool Anxiety Scale
- Screen for Child Anxiety-Related Emotional Disorders (SCARED)
- The Pediatric Anxiety Rating Scale (PARS)
- The Spence Children's Anxiety Scale
- The Youth Anxiety Measure for *DSM-5*

Adult and Older Adults Screening Tools

- Beck Anxiety Inventory
- GAD-7
- Generalized Anxiety Disorder 2-Item (GAD-2; two questions)
- HAM-A
- Panic and Agoraphobia Scale (PAS)
- Penn State Worry Questionnaire
- Severity Measure for Generalized Anxiety Disorder—Adult
- Severity Measure for Panic Disorder
- The Florida Obsessive–Compulsive Inventory
- The Yale–Brown Obsessive-Compulsive Scale (YBOCS)

Essential Facts

Central to the diagnosis of GAD are the following:

- Excessive worry about life situations (health, finances, job or academic performance, social acceptance)
- The worry is not related to another mental disorder such as:
  - Fear of having a panic attack (panic disorder)
  - Excessive worry about gaining weight (anorexia nervosa)
  - Humiliation or embarrassment (social phobia)
  - Contamination (obsessive-compulsive disorder)

RISK FACTORS FOR ANXIETY AND RELATED DISORDERS

- Behavioral inhibition
- Child abuse and neglect

- Chronic medical condition
- Female gender
- Family history of anxiety, anxiety-related disorders, or mood disorders
- History of separation, divorce, or widowed
- Personal history of anxiety or excessive worry
- Personal history of stressful life events or history of trauma
- Poor, oppressed, and lower education levels
- Substance use

CLINICAL PRESENTATION FOR CHILDREN AND ADOLESCENTS WITH ANXIETY

- Appetite changes
- Ask over and over about something they worry will happen
- Avoidance
- Complain of feeling shaky, jittery, or short of breath
- Difficulty concentrating in school
- Easily embarrassed
- Excessive worry
- Excessively shy
- Frequently feel sick to avoid school or social interactions
- Hypervigilance
- Overly afraid of what others will think or say
- Overly sensitive
- Phobias
- Reactivity such as easily crying or tantrums
- Seeks parental, caregiver, teacher, peer approval
- Sleeping difficulties and/or concerns

Essential Facts

Anxiety disorders in children can vary in presentation; therefore, it is important to assess for core symptoms. For example, children with fears and phobias such as avoidance have social anxiety disorder. Separation anxiety and other related phobias are more common in children.

CLINICAL PRESENTATION FOR OLDER ADULTS WITH ANXIETY

Older adults with anxiety-related disorders may underplay or try to normalize their behaviors as a normal part of aging or an appropriate response to expected life stressors; thus, a detailed history is essential. Anxious individuals may present with memory impairment, insomnia, weight changes, treatment-resistant pain symptoms, avoidance behaviors, increased loneliness, and fatigue (Katzman et al., 2014). Other features that may suggest anxiety include the following:

- Frequent office visits or use of medical services
- Increased dependency
- Insistent reports of pain
- Sleep or appetite changes
- Unexplained gastrointestinal symptoms

FACTORS TO CONSIDER WHEN CHOOSING TREATMENT

- Availability of cognitive behavioral therapy
- Co-occurring psychiatric and medical conditions and treatments
- Current medications
- Past treatment history
- Preferences (Koran et al., 2007).
- Severity of presenting symptoms (Koran et al., 2007).

Essential Facts

Neurologic, cardiovascular, gastrointestinal, metabolic, and vitamin deficiencies can mimic anxiety disorders.

MANAGEMENT CONSIDERATIONS

Management of anxiety involves comprehensive assessment based on a detailed patient history and collateral sources, as well as physical examination and mental-state examinations to properly establish diagnosis. Healthcare providers should consider organic causes for anxiety or medication-induced etiology. Treatment and management options for anxiety in children, adolescents, and adults depend on a combination of physiologic and emotional changes, severity of symptoms, and the individual's coping abilities (see Table 6.4). Mild to moderate anxiety may be managed with psychoeducation, family education, and psychotherapy, whereas more persistent anxiety may require a combination of pharmacotherapy and psychotherapy. Although mild anxiety is frequently described as being clinically nonsignificant, it can significantly impact emotional, social, and professional functioning. Often in early childhood, mild to moderate anxiety symptoms present as shyness or social apprehension; however, if not recognized and left untreated, these symptoms may lead to maladaptive coping and/or other psychologic conditions in adulthood.

Tests to Rule Out Organic Etiologies for Anxiety States

- Cardiovascular disorders (arrythmia)
- Complete blood count
- Fasting blood glucose levels
- Iron studies
- Lipid panel

Table 6.4

Levels of Anxiety

Anxiety Level	Sensory and Physiologic Symptoms	Cognitive and Emotional Symptoms	Example
Level 1: Mild	Heightened sensory stimulation Pupils constricted	Increased motivation Focused attention for problem-solving and protection Improves engagement in goal-directed activities	Provides focus to study
Level 2: Moderate	Disturbing or alarming feeling that something is wrong Normal vital signs Mild increase in heart rate Increased muscle tenseness and restlessness Generally, more persistent	Feelings of nervousness or agitation; restlessness Easily distracted Diminished concentration but with assistance can be redirected to process information to solve problems	Concentration difficulties at work while waiting for a family member's breast biopsy results
Level 3: Pathologic or severe	Hypervigilance Response > threat Hyper-focused with concentration on one particular detail only Headaches, palpitations, trouble falling or staying asleep Muscles tighten Sweating Vital signs increase Shortness of breath Throat tightness Sweating Pupils enlarge	Difficulties with thinking, processing, and reasoning Confusion, dread, restless, irritability, anger Primitive survival skills take over defensive responses Functional impairment that impairs well-being (personal, social, occupational) A sudden episode of intense fear that triggers severe physical reactions when the reaction is disproportionate to the level of real danger	Intense feelings of worry, self-doubt, headache, nausea, diarrhea, excessive sweating, and rapid heartbeat while engaging in social situations
Level 4: Panic	Adrenaline surge Emotional–psychomotor realm leads with accompanying fight, flight, or freeze responses Intense feeling of terror Vital signs increase Pupils enlarge	Cognitive process shuts down Inability to function or communicate Hallucinations/delusions Loss of reality Illogical thinking	Experiences panic in high places and becomes agitated and with a sensation of being unable to move or being "frozen" and requires assistance to get down safely

- Liver enzymes
- Metabolic panel
- Nutritional deficiencies
- Thyroid-stimulating hormone
- Urine toxicology for substance use

Medical Conditions to Consider in the Evaluation of Panic Attacks

- Cardiac conditions (e.g., arrhythmias or supraventricular tachycardia)
- Hyperthyroidism
- Hyperparathyroidism
- Pheochromocytoma
- Pulmonary conditions (e.g., asthma or chronic obstructive pulmonary disease)
- Vestibular dysfunctions
- Seizure disorders
- Vestibular dysfunctions

Other Lab Monitoring Considerations

- Blood pressure
  - Baseline, 1 month and with dose changes
- Body mass index (BMI)
  - Baseline, repeat 4 to 6 weeks and 6 months
- Bone mineral density
  - Baseline in older adults and follow-up as clinically indicated
- Cardiac Doppler
- Electrocardiogram (EKG)
  - Baseline and dose changes
  - Monitor children and older adults with more caution
- Electrolytes
  - Baseline, repeat 4 to 6 weeks and 6 months
  - Monitor older adults for hyponatremia with more caution
  - Assess fall risk due to hypotension
- Pregnancy test if applicable
- Screen for prevalence of potentially inappropriate medication (PIM) in older adults associated with increased morbidity, mortality, and decrease in quality of life; for example, use Screening Tool in Older Persons' Prescriptions (STOPP) Beers Criteria
- Suicidality
  - Baseline, daily, weekly, monthly, or variable depending on clinical presentation
- Thyroid tests
  - Baseline and follow-up as clinically indicated
- Urine toxicology for substance use
- Vitamin D, B_1, B_6, B_{12}, folic acid
  - Baseline and if clinically indicated

Essential Facts

When to suspect a nonpsychiatric disorder as the underlying cause of anxiety symptoms:

- The onset of anxiety symptoms first manifest when older than 35 years of age
- No personal history of anxiety (i.e., phobias, or separation anxiety in childhood)
- No reported family history of anxiety
- Absence of significant life events triggering the anxiety
- No reports of avoidance behaviors
- Lack of response to anxiolytic agents

(Chen et al., 2002)

Antidepressant medications, selective serotonin reuptake inhibitors (SSRIs), and selective norepinephrine reuptake inhibitors (SNRIs) increase the effects of serotonin and norepinephrine, which help regulate anxiety, mood, and social behavior. In general, due to their safety profile and tolerability, SSRIs and SNRIs are the first-line medication treatment for children and adults with anxiety and anxiety-related disorders; TCAs and MAOIs are generally prescribed as second-line due to their side effects and tolerability profiles (Chapter 5 discusses antidepressant use). Prescribing considerations for SSRIs and SNRIs include the following:

- Adverse effect profile
- Availability and cost
- Comorbidities
- Danger of overdose
- Past treatment response (personal and family) or side effects
- Patient and guardian preference
- Possible drug interactions
- Severity of illness

Medication in combination with psychotherapy has been shown to be highly effective for anxious individuals. Although the risk of suicidality may increase upon initiation of SSRIs in children and adolescents, the risk of not treating may negatively impact school and social functioning, leading to ongoing distress.

It is important to note that informed consent is an ongoing process; healthcare providers must have discussions about the risks, benefits, alternative management options, goals, and expectations of therapeutic options and give patients an opportunity to ask questions. Providers must also assess for social support, stigma, personal coping, and caregiver burden. Providers must conduct a thorough review and reappraisal of the diagnosis to (a) assess for possible underlying conditions and issues and (b) evaluate patient adherence and pharmacokinetic/pharmacodynamic factors and treatment plan needs if no improvement is observed after 4 to 8 weeks of treatment.

This section provides a general overview of pharmacologic agents prescribed for anxiety disorders.

Essential Facts

Duloxetine is the only U.S. Food and Drug Administration (FDA)-approved medication for children 7 years old and older diagnosed with GAD.

OVERVIEW OF MEDICATIONS FOR CHILDREN WITH GENERALIZED ANXIETY DISORDER

DULOXETINE (CYMBALTA)

- This is the only FDA-approved medication for childhood anxiety disorders.
- Other medications are used for childhood anxiety disorders but have not been FDA approved.
- "Off label" medications include sertraline, fluoxetine, fluvoxamine, paroxetine, and venlafaxine.

Drug Class

- Serotonin norepinephrine reuptake inhibitor (SNRI)

U.S. Food and Drug Administration-Approved Age

- 7 years old or older

Dosage Forms, Dosage, and Titration

- Capsule

Prescribing Considerations for Children and Adolescents for Duloxetine

- Do not open or crush the capsule; swallow whole.
- Therapeutic action may take 2 to 4 weeks.
- Peak plasma concentrations are higher in children with lower body weight.
- If activating, recommend morning doses.
- Adjust based on benefits-to-risk ratio optimization.
- May activate bipolar disorder and suicidal ideation.
- Assess growth (height and weight).
- If no response in 4 to 6 weeks, consider alternative medication and/or reassess diagnosis.
- Assess for activation, restlessness, jitteriness, hyperactivity, hypomania, or mania.
- Note there may be an increased risk for suicidal thoughts and behavior.

BENZODIAZEPINE USE IN CHILDREN

To date, no long-term studies are available for benzodiazepine use in children. Controlled trials do not support the use of benzodiazepine for treating pediatric psychiatric disorders; therefore, no firmly established indication for their use exists (Kuang et al., 2017). Although benzodiazepines are well tolerated, due to the risk of developing dependence, benzodiazepines are prescribed shortterm to alleviate more acute distress or physical symptoms (Riddle, 2015). Benzodiazepines are sometimes prescribed as a "bridge" in early treatment to (a) reduce acute anxiety symptoms before SSRIs become effective and (b) promote participation in therapy and school attendance, and resume overall functioning. Adverse effects may include dependence, daytime drowsiness and sedation, cognitive blunting, disinhibition, and behavioral agitation (Riddle, 2015).

U.S. FOOD AND DRUG ADMINISTRATION-APPROVED BENZODIAZEPINES IN CHILDREN

- **Chlordiazepoxide:** if older than 6 years of age, 5 mg every 6 to 12 hours or 10 mg every 8 to 12 hours daily
- **Diazepam:** 1 mg every 6 to 12 hours daily
- **Oxazepam:** if older than 12 years of age, 10 to 15 mg every 6 to 8 hours daily

OTHER MEDICATIONS USED TO MANAGE ANXIETY-RELATED CONDITIONS IN CHILDREN

- Alpha-agonists & Alpha Blockers (Table 6.5)

U.S. FOOD AND DRUG ADMINISTRATION INDICATION

Clonidine (Immediate-Release And Extended Release); Kapvay (Extended Release)

- FDA approved for attention deficit hyperactivity in children 6 to 17 years of age
- Adjunct or monotherapy
- Dosing extended release

Catapres, Jenloga, Duraclon (Immediate Release)

- FDA approved for hypertension in children ≥ 12 years old and older and adults
- Used "off label for anxiety in children"
- Prescriber considerations

Considerations Before Initiating Guanfacine

- Establish a baseline blood pressure.
- Monitor blood pressure throughout treatment and following dose adjustments.

Table 6.5

Other Anti-Anxiety Medications: Alpha Adrenergic Agonists & Alpha Blockers

Generic Name (Brand Name)	Dosage Forms	FDA Approval	Clinical Considerations
Prazosin (Minipress)	Capsule	*Adults:* hypertension *Off-Label:* PTSD-related nightmares and sleep disruption, benign prostate hypertrophy, Raynaud phenomenon *Pediatrics:* safety in pediatric use has not been established *Off-Label:* hypertension *Older Adult Considerations:* *	Drug Class: Alpha 1 Blocker; Antihypertensive Take at night to reduce side effects of drowsiness Monitor BP due to risk of hypotension Taper slowly to avoid rebound hypertension
Clonidine IM formulations: **Catapres** **Jenloga** **Catapres** **Duraclon** ER Formulations: **Kapvay** **Guanfacine** **Intuniv**	Injectable Solution Patch, Extended-Release Tablet, Immediate-Release Tablet, Extended-Release	*Adults:* hypertension, ADHD *Non-FDA:* migraines, opiate withdrawal, open-angle glaucoma, treating symptoms of menopause, nicotine dependence, Tourette syndrome, pain management via epidural infusion *Off-Label:* acute hypertension, EtOH withdrawal, smoking cessation, restless legs syndrome, Tourette syndrome, cyclosporine nephrotoxicity, menopausal flushing, dysmenorrhea, opioid withdrawal, post herpetic neuralgia, psychosis, pheochromocytoma diagnosis *Pediatrics:* Kapvay: attention deficit hyperactivity in children ≥ 6 years of age; adjunct or monotherapy *Older Adult Considerations:* *	Drug Class: Alpha2-Adrenergic Agonist; Antihypertensive When splitting daily dosages, larger doses are preferred to be taken at bedtime For pediatrics: Immediate release: Hypertension in children ≥ 12 years old and adults Off-label: anxiety in children Guanfacine: attention deficit hyperactivity in children ≥ 6

*Start at the lowest dosage and titrate slowly while monitoring the patient for any side effects.
ADHD, attention deficit hyperactive disorder; BP, blood pressure; ER, extended release; EtOH, ethanol alcohol; FDA, U.S. Food and Drug Administration; IM, intramuscular; PTSD, posttraumatic stress disorder

Taper Dosing

- If discontinued abruptly, there is a risk of rebound hypertension.
- Taper medication even if another medication is started; be aware of drug–drug interactions.
- When discontinuing, decrease dose by 0.1 mg every 3 to 7 days.

Guanfacine Extended Release (Intuniv)

- FDA approved for attention deficit hyperactivity in children 6 to 17 years of age
- Adjunct or monotherapy

Guanfacine Immediate Release (Tenex)

- FDA approved for hypertension in adults
- Used "off label" for anxiety in children

Prescriber Considerations Before Initiating Guanfacine

- Establish a baseline blood pressure
- Monitor blood pressure throughout treatment and following dose adjustments

Taper Dosing

- If monitored abruptly, there is a risk of rebound hypertension.
- Taper medication even if another medication is started; be aware of drug–drug interactions.
- When discontinuing, decrease dose by 0.1 mg every 3 to 7 days.

U.S. FOOD AND DRUG ADMINISTRATION APPROVED FOR OBSESSIVE-COMPULSIVE DISORDER

Fluvoxamine (Luvox Immediate Release)

- Only FDA-approved treatment for OCD in children 8 years of age and older
- Ages 8 to 17, start 25 mg at bedtime and increase by 25 mg every 4 to 7 days
- Ages 8 to 11, maximum dose 200 mg
- Ages 12 to 17, maximum dose 300 mg

Essential Facts

When starting SSRIs, SNRIs, and TCAs, some individuals experience a few mild side effects, such as feeling agitated, shaky, or anxious. These effects can be troublesome at first, but they generally improve with time. To avoid these side effects, start medication at low dosages.

Essential Facts

Risk factors for anxiety disorders include genetics, brain chemistry, personality, and life events.

Essential Facts

Escitalopram, paroxetine, venlafaxine XR, duloxetine, and buspirone are the only medications that have received FDA indication for GAD in adults.

MEDICATIONS FOR ADULTS WITH ANXIETY DISORDERS

Unlike benzodiazepines and barbiturates, buspirone (Buspar) is an anxiolytic drug with low abuse potential (see Table 6.6). Buspirone is used to manage GAD and other anxiety-related disorders or to provide short-term relief for anxiety-related symptoms. Buspirone functions as a partial agonist at 5-HT_{1A} receptors and as an antagonist at DA D_2-like receptors. Typically, it takes 2 to 4 weeks for buspirone to achieve anxiolytic effects. According to Wilson and Tripp (2020), buspirone, which is FDA approved for GAD, is considered to be as effective as benzodiazepine treatment. Buspirone's risk profile is as follows:

- Low abuse potential
- Low risk for developing physical dependence or withdrawal
- Less sedating effects compared to other anxiolytics
- No anticonvulsant or muscle-relaxing properties
- No significant interaction with central nervous system (CNS) depressants (alcohol)

ANTIHISTAMINES

Due to their quick onset of action and sedating effects, antihistamines are used for anxiety symptoms (see Table 6.7). Antihistamines are especially helpful for anxiety-induced insomnia, and, unlike benzodiazepines, antihistamines do not cause addiction.

Table 6.6

Non-Benzodiazepine Anxiolytics

Generic Name (Brand Name)	Dosage Forms	FDA Approval	Clinical Considerations
Buspirone (Buspar)	Tablet	*Adults:* GAD *Non-FDA:* augmentation for MDD *Pediatrics:* safety in pediatric use has not been established *Off-Label:* GAD *Older Adult Considerations:* *	Avoid use in patients with renal and hepatic impairments Can be dosed BID or TID Metabolized by the liver

*Start at the lowest dosage and titrate slowly while monitoring the patient for any side effects.
BID, twice a day; FDA, U.S. Food and Drug Administration; GAD, generalized anxiety disorder; MDD, major depressive disorder; TID, three times a day.

Table 6.7

Antihistamines

Generic Name (Brand Name)	Dosage Forms	FDA Approval	Clinical Considerations
Hydroxyzine (Atarax)	Tablet Capsule Syrup/Oral Suspension Injectable Solution	*Adults:* anxiety, pruritus, preoperative sedation *Off-Label:* nausea/vomiting *Pediatrics:* safety in pediatric use has not been established. *Older Adult Considerations:* no adjustment is needed	Can be useful for anxiety due to alcohol withdrawal Useful for sleep No titration generally required

FDA, U.S. Food and Drug Administration.

Essential Facts

- Due to hydroxyzine's sedating effects, it provides quick relief of symptoms.
- Consider hydroxyzine for patients who have a history of substance abuse.

BENZODIAZEPINES

Benzodiazepines are among the most widely prescribed medications for psychiatric conditions and anxiety-related disorders (see Table 6.8). Benzodiazepines have been shown to be efficacious for the treatment of anxiety disorders; however, they should be prescribed with caution for certain populations.

Essential Facts

Benzodiazepines are CNS depressants.

- When prescribing benzodiazepnes, educate and caution individuals against engaging in hazardous activities, including (a) operating machinery, (b) driving a motor vehicle, and (c) other activities requiring alertness.
- To avoid concomitant use of alcohol or other CNS-depressant drugs, consider (a) potential for tolerance (short-term rather than long-term use is preferred due to addiction potential), (b) potential for dependence, (c) risk of seizure from abrupt discontinuation, and (d) concerns about falls in older adults.

BARBITURATES

Derived from barbituric acid, barbiturates act on the CNS and have been used as sedatives or anesthetics. As a drug class, these drugs are

Table 6.8

Benzodiazepines

Generic Name (Brand Name)	Dosage Forms	FDA Approval	Clinical Considerations
Alprazolam (Xanax)	Tablet: Schedule IV Tablet Extended-Release: Schedule IV Tablet, ODT: Schedule IV Oral Solution: Schedule IV	*Adults:* GAD, social phobia, panic disorder, insomnia, status epilepticus/seizures, premedication for anesthetic procedures *Non-FDA:* agitation, alcohol withdrawal symptoms, muscle spasms, sedation, restless legs syndrome, sleepwalking disorder *Off-Label:* premenstrual syndrome, insomnia, sleep behavior disorders, somatic sympotms associated with anxiety *Pediatrics:* safety in pediatric use has not been established. *Older Adult Considerations:* *,**,***	Risks in pregnancy for cleft lip/palate and urogenital and neurologic malformations Consider synergistic effects when mixed with alcohol leading to CNS depression and death.
Chlordiazepoxide (Librax, Librium)	Capsule: Schedule IV	*Adults:* GAD, social phobia, panic disorder, insomnia, status epilepticus/seizures, premedication for anesthetic procedures *Non-FDA:* agitation, alcohol withdrawal symptoms, muscle spasms, sedation, restless legs syndrome, sleepwalking disorder *Pediatrics:* safety in pediatric use has not been established in children younger than 6 years *Older Adult Considerations*: *,**,*** Decrease the usual dose by 50%	An intramuscular dose of 50 to 100 mg can be given every 4 hours for alcohol withdrawal (not available in the U.S.).
Clonazepam (Klonopin)	Tablet Dispersible: Schedule IV Tablet: Schedule IV	*Adults:* GAD, social phobia, panic disorder, insomnia, status epilepticus/seizures, premedication for anesthetic procedures	Risks in pregnancy for cleft lip/palate and urogenital and neurologic malformations.

*Start at the lowest dosage and titrate slowly while monitoring the patient for any side effects.
**Older adult patients usually require a lower benzodiazepine dosage due to increased risk of sensitivity, risks of cognitive impairment, delirium and slower metabolism.
***Avoid in older adults concurrently taking opioids or gabapentinoids and/or with history of falls and/or fractures

(*continued*)

Table 6.8

Benzodiazepines (*continued*)

Generic Name (Brand Name)	Dosage Forms	FDA Approval	Clinical Considerations
		Non-FDA: agitation, alcohol withdrawal symptoms, muscle spasms, sedation, restless legs syndrome, sleepwalking disorder *Pediatrics:* safety in pediatric use has not been established *Older Adult Considerations:* *,**,***	Consider synergistic effects when mixed with alcohol leading to CNS depression and death.
Diazepam (Valium)	Tablet: Schedule IV Oral Solution: Schedule IV Rectal Gel: Schedule IV Injectable Solution: Schedule IV Intramuscular Device: Schedule IV	*Adults:* GAD, social phobia, panic disorder, insomnia, status epilepticus/seizures, premedication for anesthetic procedures *Non-FDA:* agitation, alcohol withdrawal symptoms, muscle spasms, sedation, restless legs syndrome, sleepwalking disorder *Pediatrics:* start at 1 mg two to four times per day and gradually increase *Older Adult Considerations:* *,**,***	Risks in pregnancy for cleft lip/palate and urogenital and neurologic malformations. Consider synergistic effects when mixed with alcohol leading to CNS depression and death.
Lorazepam (Ativan)	Tablet: Schedule IV Oral Concentrate: Schedule IV Injectable Solution: Schedule IV	*Adults:* GAD, social phobia, panic disorder, insomnia, status epilepticus/seizures, premedication for anesthetic procedures *Non-FDA:* agitation, alcohol withdrawal symptoms, muscle spasms, sedation, restless legs syndrome, sleepwalking disorder *Off-Label:* anxiolytic/sedation in ICU, chemotherapy-induced nausea/vomiting, chronic insomnia	Preferred medication in older adults due to its short-acting and inactive metabolite. Consider synergistic effects when mixed with alcohol leading to CNS depression and death.

*Start at the lowest dosage and titrate slowly while monitoring the patient for any side effects.
**Older adult patients usually require a lower benzodiazepine dosage due to increased risk of sensitivity, risks of cognitive impairment, delirium and slower metabolism.
***Avoid in older adults concurrently taking opioids or gabapentinoids and/or with history of falls and/or fractures.

(*continued*)

Table 6.8

Benzodiazepines (*continued*)

Generic Name (Brand Name)	Dosage Forms	FDA Approval	Clinical Considerations
		Pediatrics: safety in pediatric use has not been established. *Off-Label:* status epilepticus, anxiolytic/sedation/agitation, Chemotherapy-induced nausea/vomiting *Older Adult Considerations:* divided doses and titrate slowly*,**,***	
Clorazepate (Tranxene)	Tablet	*Adults:* GAD, seizures *Pediatrics:* safety in pediatric use has not been established less than 9 years 9 to 12 years partial seizures 7.5 mg BID At age 12, same dose as adults	Advise patients to use at night if taking a single dose.
Oxazepam (Serax)	Capsule: Schedule IV	*Adults:* GAD, social phobia, panic disorder, insomnia, status epilepticus/seizures, premedication for anesthetic procedures *Non-FDA:* agitation, alcohol withdrawal symptoms, muscle spasms, sedation, restless legs syndrome, sleepwalking disorder *Pediatrics:* safety in pediatric use has not been established in children younger than 6 years Children > 12 years can take 10 to 15 mg three to four times per day *Older Adult Considerations:**,**,***	Short half-life making it a drug of choice in older adults.

*Start at the lowest dosage and titrate slowly while monitoring the patient for any side effects.
**Older adult patients usually require a lower benzodiazepine dosage due to increased risk of sensitivity, risks of cognitive impairment, delirium and slower metabolism.
***Avoid in older adults concurrently taking opioids or gabapentinoids and/or with history of falls and/or fractures
BID, twice a day; CNS, central nervous system; FDA, U.S. Food and Drug Administration; GAD, generalized anxiety disorder; MDD, major depressive disorder; OCD, obsessive-compulsive disorder; ODT, orally disintegrating tablet.

no longer recommended to treat anxiety disorders because of their high potential to become addictive. Barbiturates are also dangerous in overdose because there are no good treatments to reverse a barbiturate overdose.

SELECTIVE SEROTONIN REUPTAKE INHIBITORS (SSRIs)

SSRIs and SNRIs are both first-line treatments for panic disorder, GAD, AD, and social anxiety disorder and have been shown to be efficacious for the treatment of anxiety disorders (see Tables 5.2 through 5.4 in Chapter 5 for more information).

USED FOR ANXIETY AND ANXIETY-RELATED DISORDERS

BETA BLOCKERS

Propranolol

Although not an FDA indication, propranolol responds well to anxiety by (a) blocking peripheral and central beta-adrenergic receptors and (b) reducing the autonomic hyperactivity and hyperarousal associated with anxiety increases in heart rate, blood pressure, respiration rate, tremors, and sweating. As an anxiolytic that has a quick onset of action, propranolol can be prescribed to reduce the physical symptoms that accompany performance anxiety (Ernst et al., 2016). See also Table 6.9.

Essential Facts

Propranolol has also shown to be effective with PTSD by altering how memories are stored in the brain and can have an amnestic effect on unpleasant memories (Ernst et al., 2016).

Mechanism of Action

- Competes at the receptor level with catecholamines (adrenaline and noradrenaline) to inhibit sympathetic effects.
- Blocks ß-adrenoreceptors (both beta-1 and beta-2).
- Highly lipophilic.
- Complete absorption of the drug occurs following oral administration.

U.S. Food and Drug Administration Indication

- Targets peripheral sites of the noradrenergic system to treat myocardial infarction, hypertension, coronary artery disease, and tachyarrhythmias (Ernst et al., 2016).

Table 6.9

Beta Blockers

Generic Name (Brand Name)	Dosage Forms	FDA Approval	Clinical Considerations
Propranolol (Inderal)	Oral Solution Injectable Solution Capsule, Extended Release	*Adults:* *Off-Label:* panic disorder, aggressive behavior, esophageal or variceal bleeding *Pediatrics:* safety in pediatric use has not been established *Off-Label:* hypertension, arrhythmias, hypercyanotic spells, thyrotoxicosis	Monitor BP and heart rate May cause sedation or drowsiness
Atenolol (Tenormin), Bisoprolol (Zebeta), Metoprolol (Lopressor, Toprol XL) Nadolol (Corgard), Nebivolol (Bystolic)	Tablet	*Adults:* post-myocardial infarction, angina pectoris, hypertension *Non-FDA:* cardiac dysrhythmia, congenital long QT syndrome, infantile hemangioma, migraine, postoperative cardiac complication, thyrotoxicosis *Off-Label:* alcohol withdrawal syndrome, supraventricular arrhythmias, thyrotoxicosis *Pediatrics:* safety in pediatric use has not been established *Off-Label:* hypertension *Older Adult Considerations:**	Monitor BP and heart rate

*Start at the lowest dosage and titrate slowly while monitoring the patient for any side effects.
BP, blood pressure; FDA, U.S. Food and Drug Administration.

Benefits of Propranolol in Anxiety

- Generally it is well tolerated.
- It has beneficial effects on sleep.
- It may reduce the severity of coexisting depressive symptoms.
- It reduces somatic symptom severity.
- It does not impair memory
- Reduces startle potentiation during prolonged threat periods
- Quick onset of action
- Helpful in PTSD

ANTICONVULSANTS (GABAERGIC DRUGS)

Pregabalin and Gabapentin

In clinical practice, medications not approved for anxiety are commonly used "off-label." For example, although not FDA approved as an anxiolytic, pregabalin and gabapentin are well tolerated and efficacious in reducing the severity of the acute psychologic and physical symptoms of anxiety (Baldwin & Ajel, 2007). Through their structural relationship to GABA, pregabalin and gabapentin play an important role in decreasing excitatory input (glutamate) at the receptor sites responsible for the transmission important in the psychobiology of anxiety and arousal (Sethi et al., 2005). According to Baldwin and Ajel (2007), pregabalin has comparable efficacy to certain benzodiazepines and venlafaxine (Baldwin et al., 2013).

Pregabalin (Schedule V Controlled Substance)

Mechanism of Action

- The exact mechanism of action with the GABA receptors is unknown.
- It binds with the alpha2-delta-1 site (a subunit of voltage-gated calcium channels) in CNS tissues.
- Through its effects on calcium channels, pregabalin reduces the release of glutamate, reduces the synthesis of excitatory synapses, and blocks the trafficking of new voltage-gated calcium channels to the cell surface (Baldwin et al., 2013).
- Antiepileptic effects from activity on calcium channels are used to reduce neurotransmitter release.

U.S. Food and Drug Administration Indication

Adverse Effects

- Postheraptic neuralgia
- Fibromyalgia
- Neuropathic pain
- Diabetic peripheral neuropathy
- Somnolence
- Dizziness
- Weight gain
- Potential for abuse and dependence (Schedule V)
- Requires taper to prevent withdrawal effects
- Avoid in patients with history of substance misuse due to risks of death in overdose
- In older adults increase risks associated with concurrent use with benzodiazpines and opioids (Beers Criteria, 2019, p. 12)

Benefits of Pregabalin in anxiety

- Generally it is well tolerated.
- It has beneficial effects on sleep.
- It may reduce the severity of coexisting depressive symptoms.
- It reduces somatic symptom severity.
- It does not impair memory.

Gabapentin

The anticonvulsant drug gabapentin is used to prevent seizures and to treat postherpetic neuralgia; however, due to its calming effects, gabapentin is used off-label to treat anxiety.

U.S. Food and Drug Administration Indication

- Postherpetic neuralgia
- Adjunctive to treatment of partial seizures (12 years old or older with epilepsy and 3- to 12-year-olds with partial seizures)
- Moderate-to-severe restless legs syndrome (RLS)

Mechanism of Action

- The exact mechanism of action with the GABA receptors is unknown.
- It binds with the alpha2-delta-1 site (a subunit of voltage-gated calcium channels) in CNS tissues.
- Through its effects on calcium channels, pregabalin reduces the release of glutamate, reduces the synthesis of excitatory synapses, and blocks the trafficking of new voltage-gated calcium channels to the cell surface (Baldwin et al., 2013).
- Antiepileptic effects from activity on calcium channels are used to reduce neurotransmitter release.

Adverse Effects

- Fatigue
- Dizziness
- Headache
- Taper the dose over more than 7 days to discontinue the medication

Benefits of Propranolol in Anxiety

- Mild side-effect profile
- Generally is well tolerated
- Beneficial effects on sleep
- Reduces somatic symptom severity

Essential Facts

Due to psychomotor impairment associated with benzodiazepines, caution older adults of the risk for falls and fractures.

MEASURING AND MONITORING THERAPEUTIC RESPONSE

Anxiety disorders may respond to psychologic and pharmacologic treatment but are generally not treated to remission. After treatment is started, healthcare providers should monitor change in crucial symptoms, such as frequency and intensity of distress, anxiety symptoms and/or panic attacks, level of anticipatory anxiety, degree of avoidance, and functional abilities (Koran et al., 2007). The main goal of therapy is to provide symptomatic relief and to prevent or reduce the severity and frequency of anxiety symptoms and attacks so individuals can return to their normal functioning (Sethi et al., 2005). Medications should be initiated at low doses and slowly titrated to reach optimal therapeutic effects. Patient subjective report, objective assessment findings, collateral sources, and rating scales can be used to help assess a patient's progress. According to Katzman et al. (2014), a response to therapy is often defined as a percentage reduction in symptoms (usually 25% to 50%) on an appropriate scale.

After the initial assessment, arrange a follow-up session every 2 to 4 weeks during the first 3 months of treatment and every month thereafter. Education ought to be provided on early side effects and timing to experience maximum effects of medication. For example, it may take over 2 weeks to reach the full anxiolytic effect of SSRI or SNRI medications. Additionally, risks associated with benzodiazepines should be clearly explained along with an understanding that they are intended for an as-needed basis when anxiety levels are elevated. For individuals under age 30, prescribers of SSRIs or SNRIs warn patients and family members about increased risk of suicidal thinking and self-harm. Providers arrange to see patients for an appointment within 1 week of first prescribing and monitor the risk of suicidal thinking and self-harm weekly for the first month (Katzman et al., 2014).

WHEN TO CONSULT OR REFER

Due to their broad clinical presentation, the identification and management of anxiety disorders may be challenging. Early diagnosis is important in optimizing the overall health and well-being of those affected by anxiety disorders. Refer to a specialist in cases of (a) complicating comorbidity, (b) poor response to treatment, (c) significant distress and/or functional impairment, and (d) dependent alcohol or drug misuse. In general, individuals should be treated in the least restrictive setting that is likely to be safe and effective. Hospitalization or residential treatment should be considered for individuals with a high suicide risk who pose a danger to others, are unable to perform self-care, possess co-occurring psychiatric and general medical conditions, or need intensive treatment or monitoring (Koran et al., 2007). Additionally, persistent significant symptoms of acute distress due to anxiety and/or panic despite a lengthy course of a particular treatment should trigger a reassessment of the treatment plan, including possible consultation with another qualified professional (Koran et al., 2007).

SUMMARY

To date, anxiety disorders remain a significant source of morbidity for many patients across their life span despite the presence of effective pharmacologic treatment options. The high prevalence of symptom overlap in anxiety-related disorders highlights the need for a thorough comprehensive assessment so as to increase the likelihood of accurate diagnosis. Anxiety disorders are challenging for clinicians to recognize because anxiety disorders frequently co-occur and show similarities in symptoms.

RESOURCES

National Alliance on Mental Illness (NAMI): 800-950-NAMI (800-950-6264)
Anxiety and Depression Association of America (ADAA): 240-485-1001

National Institute of Mental Health (NIMH): 866-615-6464
Centers for Disease Control and Prevention, Division of Mental Health (CDC): 800-CDC-INFO
American Psychological Association: 800-374-2721

REVIEW QUESTIONS

1. Which one of the following is the first-line therapy for children and adolescents with anxiety?
   a. SSRIs
   b. TCAs
   c. Benzodiazepines
   d. Psychotherapy
2. Risks associated with benzodiazepines include ______________.
   a. Dependence
   b. Somnolence
   c. Tolerance
   d. All of the above are correct
3. Nonbenzodiazepine anxiolytics include all of the following except ______________________.
   a. Propranolol
   b. Gabapentin
   c. Buspirone
   d. Clonazepam
4. Which one of the following statements is false?
   a. Catapres needs to be tapered when discontinuing to prevent rebound hypertension.
   b. Catapres is FDA approved for anxiety disorders in children and adults.
   c. Catapres extended release is FDA approved for attention deficit hyperactivity disorder (ADHD) in children ages 6 to 17.
   d. It is important to monitor baseline blood pressure before starting catapres in children and adults.
5. Which one of the following statements is true?
   a. Glutamate is an excitatory neurotransmitter and gamma-aminobutyric acid (GABA) is inhibitory.
   b. Glutamate is not an excitatory neurotransmitter and GABA is not inhibitory.
   c. GABA is an excitatory neurotransmitter and glutamate is inhibitory.
   d. GABA is not an excitatory neurotransmitter and GABA is not inhibitory.

REFERENCES

American Geriatrics Society Beers Criteria® Update Expert Panel (2019). American Geriatrics Society 2019 Updated AGS Beers Criteria® for Potentially Inappropriate Medication Use in Older Adults. *Journal of the American Geriatrics Society, 67*(4), 674–694. https://doi.org/10.1111/jgs.15767

American Psychiatric Association. (2013). *Diagnostic and statistical manual of mental disorders* (5th ed.). https://doi.org/10.1176/appi.books.9780890425596

Baldwin, D. S., & Ajel, K. (2007). Role of pregabalin in the treatment of generalized anxiety disorder. *Neuropsychiatric Disease and Treatment*, *3*(2), 185–191. https://doi.org/10.2147/nedt.2007.3.2.185

Baldwin, D. S., Ajel, K., Masdrakis, V. G., Nowak, M., & Rafiq, R. (2013). Pregabalin for the treatment of generalized anxiety disorder: An update. *Neuropsychiatric Disease and Treatment*, *9*, 883–892. https://doi.org/10.2147/NDT.S36453

Chen, J. P., Reich, L., & Chung, H. (2002). Anxiety disorders. *Western Journal of Medicine*, *176*(4), 249–253. https://www.ncbi.nlm.nih.gov/pmc/articles/PMC1071743

Ernst, M., Lago, T., Davis, A., & Grillon, C. (2016). The effects of methylphenidate and propranolol on the interplay between induced-anxiety and working memory. *Psychopharmacology*, *233*(19–20), 3565–3574. https://doi.org/10.1007/s00213-016-4390-y

Katzman, M. A., Bleau, P., Blier, P., Chokka, P., Kjernisted, K., Van Ameringen, M., & Canadian Anxiety Guidelines Initiative Group on behalf of the Anxiety Disorders Association of Canada/Association Canadienne des Troubles Anxieux and McGill University. (2014). Canadian clinical practice guidelines for the management of anxiety, posttraumatic stress and obsessive-compulsive disorders. *BMC Psychiatry*, *14*(Suppl. 1), Article 14. https://doi.org/10.1186/1471-244X-14-S1-S1

Koran, L. M., Hanna, G. L., Hollander, E., Nestadt, G., Simpson, H. B., & American Psychiatric Association. (2007). Practice guideline for the treatment of patients with obsessive-compulsive disorder. *American Journal of Psychiatry*, *164*(Suppl. 7), 5–53. https://psychiatryonline.org/pb/assets/raw/sitewide/practice_guidelines/guidelines/ocd.pdf

Kuang, H., Johnson, J. A., Mulqueen, J. M., & Bloch, M. H. (2017). The efficacy of benzodiazepines as acute anxiolytics in children: A meta-analysis. *Depression and Anxiety*, *34*(10), 888–896. https://doi.org/10.1002/da.22643

Reardon, T., Creswell, C., Lester, K. J., Arendt, K., Blatter-Meunier, J., Bögels, S. M., Coleman, J., Cooper, P. J., Heiervang, E. R., Herren, C., Hogendoorn, S. M., Hudson, J. L., Keers, R., Lyneham, H. J., Marin, C. E., Nauta, M., Rapee, R. M., Roberts, S., Schneider, S., ... Eley, T. C. (2019). The utility of the SCAS-C/P to detect specific anxiety disorders among clinically anxious children. *Psychological Assessment*, *31*(8), 1006–1018. https://doi.org/10.1037/pas0000700

Riddle, M. (2015). *Pediatric psychopharmacology for primary care*. American Academy of Pediatrics.

Sethi, A., Das, B. P., & Bajaj, B. K. (2005). The anxiolytic activity of gabapentin in mice. *Journal of Applied Research in Clinical and Experimental Therapeutics*, *5*(3), 415.

Subramanyam, A. A., Kedare, J., Singh, O. P., & Pinto, C. (2018). Clinical practice guidelines for geriatric anxiety disorders. *Indian Journal of Psychiatry*, *60*(Suppl. 3), S371–S382. https://doi.org/10.4103/0019-5545.224476

Wilson, T. K., & Tripp, J. (2020). Buspirone. In *StatPearls*. StatPearls Publishing. https://www.ncbi.nlm.nih.gov/books/NBK531477

7

Antipsychotic Medications

Neuroleptic or antipsychotic medications have been universally grouped according to the drugs' mechanism of action and patterns of clinical actions. The two categories of antipsychotic drugs are first-generation antipsychotics (FGAs), also known as "typical" antipsychotics, and second-generation antipsychotics (SGAs), referred to as "atypical" antipsychotics. Typical antipsychotic medication was introduced in the 1950s, and atypical antipsychotics emerged in the 1980s to reduce or alleviate psychotic symptoms and reduce the risk for psychotic relapse (Pillay et al., 2017). Psychosis *refers to a syndrome where an individual experiences a loss of contact or "break" from reality. Typically, psychotic states include hearing voices, seeing visual hallucinations, and having strange thoughts such as paranoia and/or disturbed behavior.*

In this chapter you will learn:

1. How to identify the specific manifestations of schizophrenia
2. How to compare pharmacologic options for psychotic disorders
3. How to name five key features of schizophrenia
4. How to identify screening tools for psychotic disorders
5. How to evaluate medication safety considerations in antipsychotic prescribing and management
6. How to assess therapeutic responses in psychotic disorders

Although psychosis is the hallmark symptom in schizophrenia-spectrum disorders and other psychotic disorders, psychosis can also be seen in other medical and psychiatric conditions. Antipsychotic medications remain the treatment of choice in schizophrenia-spectrum disorders because such disorders are associated with psychotic states. Psychotic states negatively impact an individual's overall functioning; therefore, psychotic states contribute to the disabling nature of these conditions (Sheffield et al., 2018).

Antipsychotic medications can vary in their effectiveness from individual to individual. In addition, typical (first generation) and atypical (second generation) antipsychotics differ in profile, and not all patients fully respond to a single antipsychotic or tolerate their side effects; in these situations, a combination of medications may be prescribed (Ortiz-Orendain et al., 2017). Often clinicians are faced with a trade-off between the benefit of alleviating psychotic symptoms and the risk of problematic, sometimes life-shortening adverse side effects, such as metabolic syndrome, obesity, type 2 diabetes mellitus, and movement disorders. These factors contribute to the challenges associated with determining which antipsychotic medication yields the best results; therefore, patient-centered treatment approaches are warranted. In most cases, a combination of pharmacotherapy and psychotherapy, in addition to patient and family psychoeducation, yields the best results. This chapter will detail psychotropic medications for use with psychotic disorders. This chapter also provides an overview of schizophrenia-spectrum disorders, screening tools, and management considerations for children and adults.

TREATMENT GOALS

The first goal of antipsychotic treatment is to (a) minimize symptoms, functional impairments (social and occupational functioning), and side effects of medication(s); (b) avoid relapses, and (c) maintain preexisting coping abilities. The second goal of antipsychotic treatment is to promote recovery, self-care, integration into society, pursuit of personal goals, and use of evidence-based psychosocial interventions.

Essential Facts

Hallucinations and delusions are both part of an altered reality. The major difference is that hallucinations are sensory and delusions are cognitive.

THE FIVE DOMAINS OF PSYCHOSIS

To consider the diagnosis for psychotic disorders, the *Diagnostic and Statistical Manual of Mental Disorders* (5th ed.; *DSM-5;* American Psychiatric Association [APA], 2013, pp. 87–90) refers to abnormalities in five distinct domains of symptomatology: (a) delusions, (b) hallucinations, (c) disorganized speech, (d) disorganized or abnormal motor behaviors including catatonic behavior, and (e) negative symptoms, which often include psychotic symptoms that present in schizophrenia-spectrum disorders (Calabrese & Al Khalili, n.d.). The psychotic symptoms associated with these symptoms are significant enough to cause distress and/or functional impairments (Sheffield et al., 2018). Additionally, it is important to note that the diagnostic process may be lengthy and take months or years due to the gradual development of symptoms (APA, 2013). Typically, the onset of psychotic symptoms or first-time schizophrenic events occurs in one's late teens or early twenties (APA, 2013).

Delusions are characterized as false beliefs: a disturbance of thinking or fixed thought patterns that are incongruent with reality. These fixed beliefs cannot be a result of an individual's culture, intelligence, or religious background. Delusion categories include grandiose, erotomanic, jealous, somatic, persecutory, mixed, or an unspecified type. *Hallucinations* are imaginary sensory perceptions. Hallucinations can include seeing imaginary objects or people, hearing voices or sounds that are not real, smelling unreal scents (olfactory hallucinations), imaginary feelings of being touched when no one is close by (tactile hallucinations), or an experience of having the sensation of taste without having eaten anything (gustatory hallucinations).

Disorganized speech is associated with communication impairment and a thought-processing disorder. Disorganized speech includes frequent derailment of speech or loose associations, incoherence, or "word salad" or tangential speech. Speech that includes frequent thought jumping, word approximations, and unclear utterances can be incomprehensible (Merrill et al., 2017). *Grossly disorganized* refers to an individual's appearance. For example, a grossly disorganized person may look disheveled or unsuitably dressed (wearing a winter coat on a hot summer day) or display inappropriate behavior. *Negative symptoms* are associated with fewer expressive emotions, poor eye contact or engagement, reduced body language and reduced interests, and reduced motivation and social participation. To diagnose schizophrenia, at least two of the five core symptoms must be present and at least one of the symptoms must be delusions, hallucinations, or disorganized speech. These symptoms must be present for at least 6 months and be causing functional impairment that cannot be attributed to another condition.

Schizophrenia is a severe mental illness that negatively impacts thoughts, decision-making, emotional processing, and management of emotions. Subcategories of schizophrenia include paranoid schizophrenia, hebephrenic schizophrenia, catatonic schizophrenia, undifferentiated schizophrenia, postschizophrenic depression, residual schizophrenia, and simple schizophrenia that is based on presenting symptomatology (Hany et al., n.d.).

Essential Facts

Alogia, or negative speech symptoms, refers to a paucity of speech expression and content; brief, empty replies.

Avolition refers to the inability to initiate or maintain goal-directed activities.

(*continued*)

Essential Facts (*continued*)

Bradyphrenia describes slowed thinking and processing of information.
Anhedonia is the decreased ability to experience pleasure or a decrease in the recollection of previously experienced pleasure.
Asociality suggests the apparent lack of interest in social interactions.

CATATONIC BEHAVIOR

Although *catatonic behavior* is often associated with schizophrenia, it is also associated with other psychologic conditions. Catatonic behavior is characterized by a combination of a psychomotor abnormality and a mood and thought disorder that includes a range of diminished reactivity in one's environment or marked apathy to rigid and purposeless motor activity. Despite being awake, an individual displays unresponsiveness to external stimuli.

Catatonia Behaviors

- **Agitation:** emotionally restless; not as a consequence of external stimuli
- **Catalepsy:** the individual upholds a fixed or frozen posture
- **Echolalia:** mimics another's speech
- **Echopraxia:** mimics another's movements
- **Grimacing:** displaying contorted facial expressions
- **Mannerism:** inflated or repetitive gestures or expressions
- **Mutism:** little to no verbal response; cannot be attributed to aphasia
- **Negativism:** opposition or unresponsiveness to external stimuli or instructions
- **Posturing:** spontaneous and active maintenance of a posture against gravity
- **Stereotypy:** repetitive movements without apparent purpose
- **Stupor:** no conscious mental activity is observed within the person's environment
- **Waxy flexibility:** slight, even resistance to bodily manipulation

Typically, there is no single cause of catatonia. Catatonia is generally associated with another mental disorder or medical condition.

Causes for Catatonia

- Abnormal neurotransmitter activity in the brain
- Idiopathic/unknown cause
- Medication side effects
- Mental or medical conditions

- Autism
- B_{12} deficiency
- Bipolar disorder
- Encephalitis
- Exposure to toxins
- Infections
- Major depressive disorder
- Neurodegenerative disease
- Psychiatric disorders
- Schizophrenia
- Severe vitamin deficiency
- Trauma

SCHIZOPHRENIA SPECTRUM AND OTHER PSYCHOTIC DISORDERS

- Brief psychotic disorder
- Catatonia (unspecified)
- Catatonia associated with another mental disorder (catatonia specifier)
- Catatonic disorder due to another medical condition
- Delusional disorder
- Psychotic disorder due to another medical condition
- Schizophrenia
- Schizophrenia spectrum (other specified) and other psychotic disorder
- Schizophrenia spectrum (unspecified) and other psychotic disorder
- Schizoaffective disorder
- Schizophreniform disorder
- Schizotypal (personality) disorder
- Substance/medication-induced psychotic disorder

Essential Facts

The origin of the word *neuroleptic*, formally known as reduce nerve functioning or tranquilize nerve function, has been derived from the Greek words for *nerve* and *affecting* (*leptikos*, meaning "seizing").

Essential Facts

Late-life psychosis or paraphrenia is a mental condition that has similar symptoms to schizophrenia but starts late in life. It encompasses delusions and visual and auditory hallucinations arising in late life.

Table 7.1

Schizophrenia Spectrum and Other Psychotic Disorders

Disorder	Key Features
Schizotypal (personality) disorder	A personality disorder that is a pervasive pattern of social and interpersonal deficits due to eccentric behavior or distorted thought patterns (suspicious and paranoid)
Delusional disorder	Main symptom is having a delusion (a false, fixed belief). The delusion lasts for at least 1 month
Brief psychotic disorder	A sudden, short period of psychotic behavior (less than a month)
Schizophreniform disorder	Psychotic symptoms for at least a month but less than 6 months
Schizophrenia	Delusions, hallucinations, behavioral changes, and functional decline that last longer than 6 months
Schizoaffective disorder	A combination of psychotic symptoms and mood symptoms (depression or bipolar disorder)
Substance/medication-induced psychotic disorder	Hallucinations, delusions, or both within a month-long period of using or withdrawing from drugs and/or alcohol
Psychotic disorder due to another medical condition	Hallucinations, delusions, or other symptoms that occur because of another illness
Catatonia associated with another mental disorder (catatonia specifier)	Diagnosis may be made when a person exhibits three or more of the diagnostic criteria for each type of catatonia.
Catatonic disorder due to another medical condition	Exhibits three or more of the diagnostic criteria for each type of catatonia; the catatonia is experienced as a result of another disorder in addition to (a) evidence that the disturbance being experienced is a direct result of another medical condition, (b) the disturbance cannot be better explained by another mental disorder, (c) the disturbance does not occur only during episodes of delirium, and (d) the disturbance causes distress or impairment in social, occupational, or other areas.
Unspecified catatonia	Symptoms of catatonia causing significant distress or impairment; however, lacks enough information or cannot be clearly attributed to another mental or medical condition.
Other specified schizophrenia spectrum and other psychotic disorder	Symptoms of hallucinations, delusions, disorganized speech, disorganized behavior, and negative symptoms that cause significant distress or impairment in important areas of functioning but do not meet full criteria for any of the primary psychotic disorders
Unspecified schizophrenia spectrum and other psychotic disorder	Symptoms presenting are characteristic of a schizophrenia spectrum and other psychotic disorder that causes clinically significant distress in areas of functioning but do not meet the full criteria for any of the disorders in the schizophrenia spectrum and other psychotic disorders diagnostic class.

DIAGNOSTIC CRITERIA FOR SCHIZOPHRENIA

According to the *DSM-5* (APA, 2013), schizophrenia is a chronic condition with an insidious onset that emerges between an individual's late teens and mid-thirties. Schizophrenia has a course of symptomology that includes the following core symptoms: delusions, hallucinations, and/or disorganized speech. Other diagnostic criteria include (a) negative symptoms and (b) declining social, occupational, or interpersonal functioning in addition to unremitting signs of disturbance and decline for at least 6 months. For an individual to be diagnosed with schizophrenia, they must have delusions or hallucinations that persist for at least 1 month (or less if being treated) and must have at least two of the following symptoms: delusions, hallucinations, disorganized speech, grossly disorganized behavior, and negative symptoms with marked difficulties in interpersonal relations, academic, or occupational functioning over a 6-month period, with at least 1 month of active phase symptoms (APA, 2013). Schizophrenia tends to have a prodromal period that is associated with difficulties in memory and attention, social withdrawal similar to depression, brief psychotic experiences, and unusual or uncharacteristic behaviors for months to years before the first psychotic episode.

Schizoaffective disorder, depression, and bipolar disorders (illnesses that include mood episodes) with psychotic qualities must be ruled out by either a negative depression screening or through verifying that the depression and/or mania has not been present for the majority of one's life. For schizoaffective disorder to be considered, the individual must experience a period of 2 weeks with positive psychotic symptoms and no mood changes. This diagnosis can only be made over an extended period of time because multiple assessments must be conducted over time. Bipolar disorder has more of a mood component whereas schizotypal personality comprises an odd pattern of behaviors that have been present over the individual's lifetime, and the odd behavior is not associated with a discrete period of time (APA, 2013).

It is important to note that not all psychosis is attributed to schizophrenia, so other conditions must be ruled out. Illnesses that can result in psychosis include mood disorder (bipolar disorder, depression), drug-induced, and other medical illnesses. Bipolar disorder has a mood component, and personality disorders present with a pattern. Individuals with schizophrenia often have poor insight into their condition; therefore, collateral information can be useful to inquire about a prodromal period or inquire about when the decline in functioning first manifested.

Essential Facts

Schizophrenia was first coined by Eugen Bleuler in 1908. The term *schizophrenia* is derived from the Greek words *schizo* (splitting) and *phren* (mind; Hany et al., n.d.).

THE SCHIZOPHRENIA HYPOTHESES

Due to schizophrenia's complexity and heterogeneity, the etiology and pathophysiologic mechanisms are not fully comprehended; however, research suggests that schizophrenia is multifactorial with several possible causes, including genetics, environment, brain chemistry, and substance use (Hany et al., n.d.). The three main hypotheses regarding the development of schizophrenia are noted in the list that follows.

1. Neurochemical hypothesis or dopamine hypothesis
   - Schizophrenia symptoms are caused by an imbalance of dopamine, serotonin, glutamate, and gamma-aminobutyric acid (GABA) on four main dopaminergic pathways.
   - Overactivation of dopamine type 2 (D2) receptors via the mesolimbic pathway is responsible for the positive symptoms (psychosis) of schizophrenia.
   - Motor symptoms of schizophrenia (extrapyramidal side effects) are caused by low levels of dopamine in the nigrostriatal pathway.
   - Negative symptoms of schizophrenia result from low mesocortical dopamine levels in the mesocortical pathway (Hany et al., n.d.).
   - The tuberoinfundibular pathway regulates prolactin secretion by the pituitary gland, and the dopamine blockade interrupts this inhibition for prolactin (gynomastia, galactorrhea, amenorrhea, sexual dysfunction).
2. Neurodevelopmental hypothesis
   - Brain anomalies or disturbances during early brain development explain the manifestations of schizophrenia.
   - The origin of schizophrenia is from disturbances of early neurodevelopment.
   - Abnormalities have been noted in the cerebral structure of individuals with schizophrenia, and an absence of gliosis suggests in-utero changes. Individuals with schizophrenia typically show motor and cognitive impairments prior to the onset of schizophrenia (Hany et al., n.d.).
   - Once first psychosis presents, imaging shows structural changes that include (a) larger ventricles, (b) smaller frontal and temporal lobes with reduced symmetry in temporal occipital and frontal lobes, and (c) decreased grey matter (Fatemi & Folsom, 2009).
   - Children who develop schizophrenia have been shown to have social and cognitive difficulties (Fatemi & Folsom, 2009).
3. Disconnection hypothesis
   - Cognitive and perceptual abnormalities seen in schizophrenia originate from specific functional disconnections expressed at the synaptic level.
   - Neuroanatomical changes seen in PET scans and functional MRI scans reveal a reduction in grey matter volume in the temporal lobe and parietal lobes.
   - Frontal lobes and the hippocampus may contribute to cognitive and memory impairments (Hany et al., n.d.).

Essential Facts

Individuals with schizophrenia have a life expectancy of 15 to 20 years shorter than the general population due to higher incidences of weight gain, diabetes, metabolic abnormalities, sedentary lifestyles, cardiovascular disease, and chronic respiratory conditions (Health Quality Ontario, 2018; National Institute for Health and Care Excellence [NICE], 2015).

SCREENING TOOLS FOR SCHIZOPHRENIA

Screening scales remain the primary method of assessing, diagnosing, and monitoring the severity of positive and negative symptoms and tracking treatment responses. Due to high suicide risk among individuals with schizophrenia, suicide assessments should be conducted routinely. The following is a list of screening scales used in the assessment, diagnosis, and monitoring of schizophrenia:

- Abnormal Involuntary Movement Scale (AIMS)
- Brief Negative Symptom Scale
- Brief Psychiatric Rating Scale
- Bush Francis Catatonia Rating Scale
- Clinical Assessment Interview for Negative Symptoms
- Clinical Global Impression Schizophrenia
- Dyskinesia Identification System Condensed User Scale (DISCUS)
- Negative Symptom Assessment-16
- Positive and Negative Symptoms Scale
- Scale for the Assessment of Negative Symptoms (SANS)
- Scale for the Assessment of Positive Symptoms

RISK FACTORS FOR SCHIZOPHRENIA AND RELATED DISORDERS

The following are risk factors for schizophrenia and related disorders:

- Issues with autoimmune system
- Complications during pregnancy or birth
  - Abnormal fetal development and low birth weight
  - Gestational diabetes
  - Preeclampsia
  - Emergency cesarean section and other birthing complications
  - Maternal malnutrition and vitamin D deficiency
- Drug use during adolescence and early adulthood
- Exposure to toxins (lead exposure)
- External stressors
- Genetics
- Male gender
- Older aged father
- Urbanicity
- Viral infection

CLINICAL ASSESSMENT OF SCHIZOPHRENIA

Schizophrenia is based on the diagnostic interview and is basically a diagnosis of exclusion. To rule out other possible causes of psychosis, it is necessary to obtain a thorough medical and psychiatric history that is supplemented by collateral information. A thorough assessment includes obtaining information about a patient through a variety of methods, face-to-face interviews, reviews of medical records, physical examinations, diagnostic testing, and history taking from other sources (Addington et al., 2017). It is beneficial to obtain as much information as possible about the patient's clinical presentation prior to the evaluation.

Essential Facts

- The lifetime risk for suicide among people with schizophrenia is about 5% (Addington et al., 2017).
- Suicide risk factors include comorbid depressive disorders, previous attempts, drug misuse, agitation or motor restlessness, fear of mental disintegration, and poor adherence to treatment (Addington et al., 2017).

Medical History

- Assessment of financial status, housing, and support network
- Assessment of suicide risk at the initial assessment, and reassessments should be ongoing
- Detailed pregnancy history
- Early childhood and development
- Family history
- Monitor for coexisting mental health conditions (depression, anxiety, and substance misuse), with regular monitoring thereafter
- Occupational, academic, and social functioning (child, adolescent, and current)
- Personal medical history and developmental history
- Prescribed medication use
- Substance use (tobacco, alcohol, marijuana, hallucinogens, stimulants, opioids, and other drugs)
- Travel history

Essential Facts

Unremarkable children who are later diagnosed with schizophrenia in adulthood may be described by family members as physically clumsy and emotionally aloof children.

Assessment of Substance Use

- Duration of past and current levels of use
- Impact on medication adherence
- Initial urine toxicology, routinely administered
- Level of dependence
- Prior treatment approaches (successful and unsuccessful approaches)
- Quantity, frequency, and patterns of substance usage
- Readiness to change
- Route of administration of substance use
- Substance(s) usage

Essential Facts

Clozapine, an SGA, has been shown to reduce suicide attempts in individuals with high-risk schizophrenia and schizoaffective disorder (Meltzer et al., 2003).

MEDICAL CONSIDERATIONS FOR PSYCHOSIS

Laboratory testing to ruleout other physical conditions includes the following:

- B_{12} levels
- Blood ethanol level
- Blood glucose level
- Complete blood count with differential
- Complete metabolic panel
- Copper levels
- HIV/syphilis serology
- Imaging studies (computed tomography [CT] head/MRI)
- Kidney functioning tests
- Liver tests
- Other serum markers (metals, etc.)
- Thyroid-stimulating hormone
- Twenty-four-hour cortisol collection; both hypercortisolism (Cushing syndrome) and adrenocortical insufficiency (Addison disease)
- Twenty-four-hour catecholamine/5-HIAA collection
- Urine toxicology screen

Essential Facts

At the time of the first psychotic episode, neuroimaging with CT or MRI can be conducted based on specific details of the patient's history, neurologic examination, or neuropsychologic testing results (Addington et al., 2017). This imaging should be done on a case-by-case basis.

Table 7.2

Medical Considerations for Psychosis

Type	Key Features
Cancer	Brain tumor or other malignancies; central nervous system neoplasm; pheochromocytoma/carcinoid syndrome
Endocrine	Adrenal insufficiency, adrenocortical insufficiency (Addison disease), hypercortisolism (Cushing syndrome), hypoglycemia, hypoparathyroidism or hyperparathyroidism, thyroid disorder
Medication and other medical condition disorders	Antiviral medications, barbiturate withdrawal, cocaine/methamphetamine abuse, digoxin, drug induced, electrolyte disorders (delirium), EtOH (Ethanol) withdrawal, heavy metal poisoning, human immunodeficiency virus (HIV), infections, marijuana, metabolic disorders, neurosyphilis phencyclidine (PCP), psychedelic intoxication, steroid use, stimulants, systemic lupus erythematosus, Wilson's disease
Neurologic	Dementia (parkinsonian features), Lewy body dementia, seizure disorders, types of encephalitis
Psychiatric disorders	Bipolar disorder, posttraumatic stress disorder, traumatic brain injury

GENERAL CONSIDERATIONS FOR TREATMENT

FGA contraindications include the following:

- Cardiomyopathy or arrythmias
- Concomitant use of anticholinergic medication
- Concomitant use of central nervous system depressants (barbiturates, opioids)
- History of hypotension
- History of severe allergy
- History of tardive dyskinesia
- Narrow-angle glaucoma
- Prostate hypertrophy
- Seizure disorder
- Additional management considerations:
  - Adverse effect profile
  - Co-occurring psychiatric and medical conditions and treatments
  - Cost and availability of resources
  - Current medication, drug–drug interactions, and side effects
  - Danger of overdose
  - Family history of heart disease (premature sudden cardiac death or prolonged QT interval, or others)
  - Past treatment history (pleasant and unpleasant subjective experiences)
  - Past treatment response (personal and family) or side effects
  - Personal, family preferences, guardian preference (Koran et al., 2007)
  - Severity of illness
  - Timing of therapeutic effect

Essential Facts

Metabolic Syndrome

Diagnosis requires three or more of the following:

- Blood pressure of 130/85 or greater
- Triglycerides of 150 or greater
- High-density lipoprotein of less than 40 in men and less than 50 in women
- Fasting blood sugar of 100 or greater
- Waist circumference of 40 inches or more in men and 35 inches or more in women

MEDICATION MANAGEMENT CONSIDERATIONS BASELINE DATA

- Assessment of nutritional status
- Cardiomyopathy
- Electrocardiogram (EKG)
- Fasting blood glucose
- Glycosylated hemoglobin (HbA1c)
- Level of physical activity
- Lipid profile
- Prolactin levels
- Vital signs, pulse, and blood pressure
- Waist and hip circumferences
- Weight and height (growth charts)

Essential Facts

The 11 indications for antipsychotic (neuroleptics) medications:

- Schizophrenia
- Bipolar disorder
- Major depressive disorder (use as adjunctive therapy)
- Tourette syndrome
- Severe behavioral problems
- Hyperactivity
- Anxiety
- Hiccups
- Acute intermittent porphyria
- Nausea/vomiting
- Tetanus

Individuals with schizophrenia who use antipsychotic medications as the mainstay of treatment require long-term treatment. Antipsychotic monotherapy should be the preferred treatment approach (Hasan et al., 2012). Because antipsychotic use is linked to adverse effects on physical health, individuals with schizophrenia require vigilant monitoring of side effects. It is important to note that informed consent is an ongoing process; healthcare providers must have discussions about the risks, benefits, alternative management options, goals, and expectations of therapeutic options and give patients and caregivers the opportunity to ask questions. Clinicians must also assess for social support, stigma, personal coping, financial situation, and caregiver burden. Providers must conduct a thorough review and reappraisal of the diagnosis to (a) assess for possible underlying conditions, comorbid conditions, and other issues; and (b) evaluate patient's adherence barriers and abilities, pharmacokinetic or pharmacodynamic factors, and treatment plan needs.

Essential Facts

Earlier onset of schizophrenia-spectrum disorders in children and young individuals appears to be associated with poorer long-term outcomes (NICE, 2015).

Antipsychotic-Associated Side Effects

Agranulocytosis is a serious side effect. Antipsychotic-associated side effects include constipation, decreased interest in sex, difficulty thinking or concentration, dizziness, dysmenorrhea, endocrine galactorrhea, extrapyramidal symptoms (EPS; akathisia/parkinsonism; tardive dyskinesia), glucose abnormalities, hypotension, insomnia, lipid abnormalities, metabolic symptoms, neuroleptic malignant syndrome (NMS), prolactin elevation, QT prolongation, restlessness, sedation, seizures, sexual dysfunction, sleepiness, and weight gain.

Neuroleptic Malignant Syndrome

The exact cause for NMS is unknown, and there are no universally accepted criteria. NMS is a rare but potentially adverse and fatal reaction to a dopamine receptor blockade that is triggered by antipsychotic drugs. NMS is

Table 7.3

Extrapyramidal Side Effects and Key Features

Akathisia	Feeling of restlessness and need to move
Akinesia	Absence of movement; loss of ability to move muscles voluntarily
Dystonia	Involuntary muscle contractions that cause slow, repetitive movements or abnormal postures
Pseudo Parkinson's	Conditions that mimic Parkinson's disease
Tardive dyskinesia	Repetitive, involuntary, abnormal movements of the face, mouth, tongue, jaw, and body (i.e., tongue protrusion, side-to-side movement of the jaw, lip smacking, puckering and pursing, and rapid eye blinking, as well as movements of the arms, legs, and trunk)

a neurologic emergency and must be managed quickly. Although there is greater risk for NMS with FSAs, cases have shown that SGAs, antiemetics, and other drugs have also caused NMS due to their dopamine-blocking properties (Berman, 2011). NMS typically develops within the first 14 days of treatment; however, it can manifest after a single dose or after many years even if the treatment and dose are constant (Berman, 2011). NMS's presentation can vary; however, NMS is often characterized by a triad of symptoms: (a) fever, (b) muscle rigidity, and (c) altered mental status (APA, 2013).

Clinical symptoms of NMS include the following:

- Abnormal reflexes
- Altered mental status, confusion
- Autonomic instability
  - Cardiac dysrhythmias
  - Diaphoresis
  - Flushing
  - Irregular pulse
  - Labile blood pressure
  - Skin pallor
  - Tachycardia
  - Tachypnea
- Blood test results
  - Acute renal failure
  - Electrolyte abnormalities
  - Elevated creatine
  - Elevated blood urea nitrogen levels
  - Elevated creatine phosphokinase
  - Elevated lactate dehydrogenase
  - Elevated liver transaminases
  - Elevated myoglobinuria
  - Iron deficiency
  - Leukocytosis
  - Metabolic acidosis
  - Rhabdomyolysis
- Dysphagia
- Extreme agitation
- Hyperpyrexia (hyperthermia)
- Incontinence
- Muscle rigidity/dystonia
- Mutism
- Seizures
- Sialorrhea

Conditions that mimic NMS include the following:

- Agitated delirium
- Drug toxification
  - Amphetamines
  - Anticholinergic
  - Cocaine
  - Methamphetamine

- Lithium
- Serotonin syndrome

- Drug-induced extrapyramidal symptoms
- Heat stroke
- Encephalopathies
- Infections (central nervous system, sepsis)
- Meningitis
- Status epilepticus
- Withdrawal syndromes (alcohol and benzodiazepine)

Clinical management of NMS can include the following strategies:

- Blood pressure control
- Cooling measures (antipyretics; cooling blankets)
- Hospitalization
- Hydration
- Immediate discontinuation of antipsychotic drug(s)
- Medical monitoring
- Medications: dopamine agonists (dantrolene, amantadine, bromocriptine); heparin (prevent thromboembolism)
- Symptomatic treatment
- Treatment of any other concurrent medical problems

Essential Facts

Auditory hallucinations; thought withdrawal, insertion, or interruption; thought broadcasting; somatic hallucinations; delusional perception; and feelings or actions controlled by external agents are "first-rank" symptoms associated with schizophrenia (Addington et al., 2017)

FIRST-GENERATION AND SECOND-GENERATION ANTIPSYCHOTICS MECHANISM OF ACTION

Chlorpromazine, an first-generation antipsychotic medication (FGA), was the first antipsychotic medication that was developed in the early 1950s (Abou-Setta et al., 2012). Antipsychotic medications have a high dopaminergic receptor-blocking power; therefore, they can cause side effects such as extrapyramidal movement disorders and irreversible tardive dyskinesia (NICE, 2013). In contrast, second-generation antipsychotic medications (SGAs) have mixed dopaminergic- and serotonergic-blocking properties. Both FGAs and SGAs are dopamine-receptor antagonists; however, SGAs also antagonize D2 dopamine receptors and have serotonin 5-HT2A and 5-HT1A receptor antagonism action (Abou-Setta et al., 2012).

SGAs also minimize FGAs' side effects, which include sedation, hypotension, weight gain, and sexual dysfunction (Abou-Setta et al., 2012). FGAs and SGAs improve tic disorders, disruptive and aggressive behaviors, schizophrenia, and behavioral disorders or irritability associated with autism. FGAs like phenothiazine derivatives can vary in their dopamine (D1–D5), histamine, and cholinergic receptor antagonism action (Abou-Setta et al., 2012). An FGA's action is primarily on the dopaminergic system and is thus effective against the positive symptoms of schizophrenia; however, FGAs have been considered to be ineffective in treating negative symptoms. FGAs that block the D2 receptors lead to EPS (e.g., tremor, slurred speech, akathisia, dystonia, tardive dyskinesia, etc.), which can vary in severity and timing of onset; therefore, vigilant monitoring is required (Abou-Setta et al., 2012).

Essential Facts

If a diagnosis of psychosis is unclear but suspected, regularly monitor (a) severity and frequency of symptoms, (b) levels of impairment and/or distress, and (c) the degree of family concern for up to 3 years (NICE, 2013).

Essential Facts

After discontinuing antipsychotic therapy, individuals should be screened for diabetes for at least 1 year due to an increased risk of type 2 diabetes after discontinuing the medication.

Table 7.4

Mechanism of Action

Typical (First-Generation Antipsychotics)	Atypical (Second-Generation Antipsychotics)
Dopamine receptor antagonists	Serotonin-dopamine antagonists: blocks D2 dopamine receptors and has serotonin 5-HT2A and 5-HT1A receptor antagonism action
Noradrenergic, cholinergic, and histaminergic blocking action (H1 histamine)	Antidepressant actions/serotonin and/or norepinephrine reuptake inhibition
Treat positive symptoms of schizophrenia (hallucinations, delusions) and decrease episodes of psychosis and relapse	Treat positive symptoms (hallucinations, delusions) and negative symptoms of schizophrenia (withdrawal, tiredness, ambivalence, apathy, and loss of emotion) and reduce relapse
Available in IV formulation	No IV formulation available
High risk of EPS and tardive dyskinesia	Fewer EPS and tardive dyskinesia instances
Risk of NMS is greater with FGAs	Risk of NMS is lower with SGAs
FDA boxed warning: higher mortality risk in older adult patients with dementia-related psychosis	FDA boxed warning of increased incidence of stroke in older adult patients with dementia

EPS, extrapyramidal symptoms; FDA, U.S. Food and Drug Administration; IV, intravenous; NMS, neuroleptic malignant syndrome

LIST OF FIRST-GENERATION ANTIPSYCHOTIC MEDICATIONS AND U.S. FOOD AND DRUG ADMINISTRATION INDICATIONS FOR POPULATIONS YOUNGER THAN 18 YEARS

- Chlorpromazine: hyperactivity, combative or explosive behaviors
- Droperidol: no FDA indication in pediatric population
- Haloperidol: no FDA indication in pediatric population
- Molindone: no FDA indication in pediatric population
- Perphenazine: no FDA indication in pediatric population
- Pimozide: Tourette syndrome, moderate, severe
- Thioridazine: no FDA indication in pediatric population
- Thiothixene: no FDA indication in pediatric population
- Trifluoperazine: no FDA indication in pediatric population

FIRST-GENERATION ANTIPSYCHOTIC USE IN CHILDREN AND ADOLESCENTS 18 YEARS OF AGE OR YOUNGER

Initially SGAs and mood stabilizers are preferred, and FGAs are more commonly prescribed in refractory or complex cases (Pillay et al., 2017).

Chlorpromazine (Thorazine)

- Approved for children ages 1 to 12 years old
- Hyperactivity with conduct disorders (combative or explosive behavior)
- Severe behavioral disorders

Dosage Forms

- Tablets
- Vial for IM injection

Haloperidol (Haldol; Haldol Decanoate)

U.S. Food and Drug Administration Approved

- Tourette disorder (used for severe, treatment-refractory cases)
- No FDA indication for children and therefore used off-label for sedation, behavioral problems, schizophrenia, and psychosis

Dosage Forms

- Tablets
- Oral concentrate liquid
- Injectable vial

Pimozide (Orap)

U.S. Food and Drug Administration Approved

- Tourette disorder, moderate to severe in those older than 8 years old

Dosage

- Tablets
- To avoid withdrawal symptoms, discontinue slowly

PRESCRIBING CONSIDERATIONS FOR CHILDREN AND ADOLESCENTS WITH FIRST-GENERATION ANTIPSYCHOTICS

- Anticholinergic effects
  - Dry mouth
  - Constipation
  - Confusion
  - Agitation
  - Xerostomia
- Endocrine
  - Gynecomastia
  - Galactorrhea
  - Menstrual problems for girls
  - Erectile dysfunction
  - Priapism
- Hematologic
  - Agranulocytosis
  - Leukopenia
  - Thrombocytopenia
  - Jaundice
- Metabolic side effects
  - Weight gain
  - Elevated glucose
  - Insulin resistance
  - Elevated cholesterol and triglycerides
  - Cardiovascular problems (torsades de pointes)
- Neurologic
  - Tardive dyskinesia
  - Akathisia
  - Dystonia
  - Tremor
  - Seizure
  - NMS
  - Photosensitivity
- Sedation and daytime sedation

Essential Facts

Chlorpromazine is prescribed to treat intractable hiccups, nausea and vomiting, acute intermittent porphyria, and may be used as part of a course of treatment for tetanus.

SECOND-GENERATION ANTIPSYCHOTIC USE FOR CHILDREN AND ADOLESCENTS WHO ARE 18 YEARS OF AGE OR YOUNGER

SGAs are first-line drugs due to having a lower risk of extrapyramidal symptoms; however, SGAs are associated with more weight gain, lipid abnormalities, and insulin resistance (Pillay et al., 2017).

LIST OF SECOND-GENERATION ANTIPSYCHOTIC MEDICATIONS AND U.S. FOOD AND DRUG ADMINISTRATION INDICATIONS FOR POPULATION AGES YOUNGER THAN 18 YEARS

- Aripiprazole: irritability associated with autism disorder, bipolar disorder, schizophrenia
- Asenapine: safety and efficacy not established in children
- Clozapine: safety and efficacy not established in children
- Iloperidone: safety and efficacy not established in children
- Lurasidone: safety and efficacy not established in children
- Olanzapine: schizophrenia, bipolar disorder/acute mania
- Paliperidone: schizophrenia
- Quetiapine: schizophrenia, bipolar disorder/acute mania
- Risperidone: schizophrenia, bipolar disorder, irritability associated with autism
- Lurasidone: safety and efficacy not established in children
- Ziprasidone: safety and efficacy not established in children

Risperidone (Risperdal, Risperdal, CONSTA, Perseris)

U.S. Food and Drug Administration Approval

- Children and adolescents
- Thirteen years and older for schizophrenia
- Ten years and older for bipolar mania
- Five years and older for irritability associated with autism

Dosage Forms

- Tablets
- Orally disintegrating tablet (ODT)*
- Liquid
- IM, depot (CONSTA)**
- Perseris is a long-acting form (SQ)**

---

*ODT can be used as an alternative for individuals who have difficulty swallowing tablets.

**Efficacy of IM and SQ dose is not established in those younger than 18 years of age.

Aripiprazole (Abilify)

U.S. Food and Drug Administration Approval

- Schizophrenia in those 13 years old and older
- Bipolar mania/acute mania in those 10 years old and older
- Tourette disorder in those 6 years old and older
- Autism associated with irritability in those 6 years old and older
  - Increase dose in 7-day increments until desired effect is achieved.

Dosage Forms

- Tablet
- ODT*
- Oral solution

Olanzapine (Zyprexa, Symbyax, Zyrexa Relprevv [Olanzapine Pamoate])

U.S. Food and Drug Administration Approval

- Schizophrenia in those 13 years old and older
- Bipolar mania/acute mania in those 13 years old and older

Dosage Forms

- Oral tablets
- ODT*
- IM
- Depot
  - Safety not established in those younger than 18 years old
- Combination olanzapine-fluoxetine capsule:
  - Safety is not established in those younger than 18 years old.

Paliperidone (Invega, Invega Sustenna, Invega Trinza, Xeplion, Trevicta)

U.S. Food and Drug ADministration Approval

- Schizophrenia in those 12 years old and older

Dosage Forms

- Extended-release oral tablets
- One-month IM injection
  - Prior to initiation of monthly IM therapy, tolerability should be established with oral paliperidone or oral risperidone.
- Three-month IM injection:
  - Efficacy of IM dose is not established in those younger than 18 years of age.
  - Prior to initiation of monthly IM therapy, tolerability should be established with oral paliperidone or oral risperidone.

---

*ODT can be used as an alternative for individuals who have difficulty swallowing tablets.

Special Considerations for Paliperidone

- Use with caution for individuals with preexisting gastrointestinal-narrowing disorders or gastrointestinal-tract alterations because drug is contained in a nondeformable controlled-release formulation.
- Swallow capsule and avoid crushing or chewing medication to avoid rapid bioavailability of paliperidone.
- Following drug release/absorption, the shell is expelled in stool.

Quetiapine (Seroquel, Seroquel XR)

U.S. Food and Drug Administration Approval

- Schizophrenia in those 13 years old and older

Dosage Forms

- Immediate release:
  - Continue therapy at lowest dose needed to maintain remission.
- Extended release:
  - Continue therapy at lowest dose needed to maintain remission.
- Bipolar disorder/ acute mania in those 10 years old or older
  - Immediate-release tablets:
    - Continue therapy at lowest dose needed to maintain remission.
  - Extended-release tablets:
    - Continue this dose dependent on clinical response.
    - Continue therapy at lowest dose needed to maintain remission.
- How to switch from immediate release to extended release:
  - Convert from immediate-release to extended-release tablets at the equivalent total daily dose and administer once daily.
  - Assess for individual dosage adjustments that may be required.

Special Considerations for Quetiapine

- If Quetiapine has been discontinued:
  - If more than 1 week discontinued, retitrate using the initial dosing schedule.
  - If less than 1 week discontinued, restart on their previous maintenance dose.
- Extended-release formulation: Do not break, chew, or crush
  - Swallow whole since drug is sustained release.

Dosage Forms

- Tablets (immediate release)
- Extended-release tablets:
  - Avoid chewing or crushing; swallow whole because Seroquil XR is controlled release.

Prescribing Considerations Children and Adolescents for Second-Generation Antipsychotics

- Injectable formulations are not approved in children/adolescents.
- Monitor weight at baseline and every 3 months ongoing.

- Screen for personal and family history of diabetes, obesity, blood pressure, fasting plasma glucose, fasting lipid profile, dyslipidemia, waist circumference, hypertension, and cardiovascular disease.
- Monitor absolute neutrophil count (stop if below 1,000/mm^3).
- Assess for tardive dyskinesia.
- If mild side effects, wait to see tolerance and determine risk versus benefit of continuing the medication.

LIST OF FIRST-GENERATION ANTIPSYCHOTIC MEDICATIONS AND U.S. FOOD AND DRUG ADMINISTRATION INDICATIONS FOR ADULT POPULATIONS

- Chlorpromazine (Thorazine): schizophrenia, agitation/aggression (severe, acute) associated with psychiatric disorders (schizophrenia, bipolar disorder, behavioral and conduct disorders), bipolar disorder, acute manic episodes (acute psychosis), nausea, vomiting, acute intermittent, porphyria, tetanus, intractable or prolonged hiccups
- Fluphenazine (Prolixin): psychotic disorders
- Haloperidol (Haldol): psychosis, schizophrenia, behavioral disorders, nonpsychotic and hyperactivity, Tourette syndrome/tic management
- Loxapine (Loxitane): schizophrenia, agitation concomitant with schizophrenia or bipolar I disorder
- Perphenazine (Trilafon): schizophrenia, nausea/vomiting in adults
- Pimozide (Orap™): Tourette disorder
- Thioridazine (Mellaril): schizophrenia
- Thiothixene (Navane): schizophrenia
- Trifluoperazine (Stelazine): schizophrenia

PRESCRIBING AND MONITORING CONSIDERATIONS

Baseline information:

- Blood pressure
- Body mass index (BMI)
- Complete blood count
- Electrocardiogram
- Fasting glucose
- Lipid profile
- Personal history and family history
- Transaminases
- Waist circumference
- Four weeks / 8 weeks, and then every 12 weeks annually

Three months:

- Blood pressure
- BMI
- Fasting glucose

- Lipid profile
- Waist circumference

Annually:

- Blood pressure
- Fasting glucose
- Lipid profile
- Waist circumference

Cigarette Smoking

Smoking prevalence for schizophrenic patients is higher than it is for the general population. Due to the high frequency of smoking in schizophrenic patients, clinicians need to check smoking status in each patient. Smoking stimulates dopaminergic activity in the brain. Cigarettes increase the activity of CYP1A2 enzymes, thus decreasing the concentration of many antipsychotics primarily metabolized by CYP1A2. Therefore, schizophrenic patients who smoke may require higher dosages of antipsychotics than nonsmokers. Upon smoking cessation, smokers may require a reduction in the dosage of antipsychotics.

Prolactin Levels

Clinicians should routinely ask people taking FGAs screening questions about symptoms of elevated prolactin.

- For women: clinicians should inquire about changes in menstruation or libido, and whether they have noticed any milk discharge from breasts.
- For men: inquiries should be made about libido and sexual dysfunction.
- Clinicians should order prolactin levels if screening questions indicate possible hyperprolactinemia.

TREATMENT OF EXTRAPYRAMIDAL SYMPTOMS

1. **Benztropine** (Cogentin)

   FDA approval: EPS and drug-induced parkinsonism (dopamine D2 receptor blocking agents)

   Mechanism of action—how a drug produces an effect in the body (MOA): reduces acetylcholine action at muscarinic receptors caused by dopamine inhibition

   Older adult: Beers Criteria as a potentially inappropriate medication to be avoided in patients 65 years and older due to its highly anticholinergic properties (The 2019 American Geriatrics Society [AGS] Beers Criteria Update Expert Panel, 2019)
2. **Deutetrabenazine** (Austedo)

   MOA: Unknown, hypothesized that (alpha-dihydrotetrabenazine [HTBZ] and beta-HTBZ) act as reversible inhibitors of the monoamine transporter type 2 (VMAT-2) and decrease the uptake of monoamines (dopamine, serotonin, norepinephrine, and histamine) into synaptic vesicles and deplete the monoamine supply.

   FDA indication: treatment of tardive dyskinesia in adults; treatment of chorea associated with Huntington disease in adults

   Dosing forms: tablets

Dietary considerations: Administer with food.

Monitor: electrolytes; EKG; signs/symptoms of worsening depression or suicidality or changes in behavior; signs and/or symptoms of NMS, restlessness, and agitation

3. **Valbenazine** (Ingrezza)

   MOA: Unknown, hypothesized that it works through the reversible inhibition of vesicular monoamine transporter 2 (VMAT2), a transporter that regulates monoamine uptake from the cytoplasm to the synaptic vesicle for storage and release.

   FDA indication: treatment of adults with tardive dyskinesia

   Dosing forms: capsule

   Dietary considerations: Administer with or without food.

   Monitor: AIMS or DISCUS

4. **Lower dose of medication**
5. **Intermittent "drug holidays"**
6. **Discontinue and change medication**

LIST OF SECOND-GENERATION ANTIPSYCHOTIC MEDICATIONS AND INDICATIONS FOR ADULT POPULATIONS

- Aripiprazole (Abilify)
- Asenapine (Saphris)
- Clozapine (Clozaril)
- Iloperidone (Fanapt)
- Lurasidone (Latuda)
- Olanzapine (Zyprexa)
- Paliperidone (Invega)
- Quetiapine (Seroquel)
- Risperidone (Risperdal)
- Ziprasidone (Geodon)

Essential Facts

Aripiprazole is recommended for the treatment of schizophrenia in individuals aged 15 to 17 years who are intolerant of or unable to take risperidone, or if schizophrenia symptoms are inadequately controlled with risperidone (NICE, 2013).

Essential Facts

In patients with poor medication adherence and high risk of illness relapses, consider long-acting injectable antipsychotic medications.

Clozapine: Special Considerations in Prescribing, Monitoring, and Management

Clozapine is FDA approved for the treatment of treatment-resistant schizophrenia and schizoaffective disorder after adequate trials of at least two other antipsychotic medications (at least one FGA; Remington et al., 2017). Dosing for clozapine must be carefully titrated to minimize the severity of adverse effects. Side effects are the potential reasons for clozapine discontinuation along with its associated risk of life-threatening leukopenia or agranulocytosis; therefore, prior to prescribing Clozaril, a baseline antinuclear antibody (ANA) must be obtained along with other screening tests. A baseline of 1,500/uL is required for the general population and a minimum of 1,000/uL for individuals with benign ethnic neutropenia (Clozapine Risk Evaluation and Mitigation Strategy [REMS], n.d.). The FDA has mandated requirements for routine monitoring and registry reporting of neutrophil counts for the duration that clozapine is administered (Clozapine REMS, n.d.). All manufacturers use one registry: the Clozapine REMS Program (Clozapine REMS, n.d.).

Essential Facts

Clozapine: White blood cell (WBC) monitoring protocol:

- Weekly during the first 6 months of administration
- Every other week for the second 6 months

Every 4 weeks after 1 year and ongoing throughout the length of treatment.

Clozapine Side Effects

- Cardiomyopathy
- Diabetes mellitus, diabetic ketoacidosis, diabetic hyperosmolar coma
- ECG changes (QT prolongation, tachycardia, atrial flutter)
- Fever
- Gastrointestinal obstruction
- Liver enzyme elevation
- Myocarditis
- Neuroleptic malignant syndrome
- Neutropenia or agranulocytosis
- Seizures
- Syncope
- Thrombocytopenia

OLDER ADULT CONSIDERATIONS

Antipsychotics are identified in the Beers Criteria (The 2019 AGS Beers Criteria Update Expert Panel, 2019) as potentially inappropriate medications to be avoided in individuals 65 years of age and older due to an increased risk of cerebrovascular accidents and an increased rate of cognitive decline and mortality in patients diagnosed with dementia. Although antipsychotics may be appropriate for schizophrenia, bipolar disorder, other mental health conditions, or short-term use as an antiemetic, they should be given in the lowest effective dose for the shortest duration possible. Antipsychotics should be used with caution in older adults due to their ability to cause or exacerbate syndrome of inappropriate antidiuretic hormone secretion (SIADH) or hyponatremia; monitor sodium closely with initiation or dosage adjustments in older adults (The 2019 AGS Beers Criteria Update Expert Panel, 2019).

Dexmedetomidine (IGALMI) is the first FDA approved sublingual alpha-2 adrenergic receptor agonist indicated in adults for the acute treatment of agitation associated with schizophrenia or bipolar I or II disorder. Currently, no pharmacologic treatment is approved for agitation or dementia-related psychosis; however, due to their major determinants of poor quality of life, SGAs are frequently prescribed off-label despite their safety concerns. Due to FGAs and SGAs' risk profile in older adults, they are to be avoided and only considered with extreme caution if the benefits outweigh the risks of treatment. For individuals with dementia, treatment for agitation and/or psychotic symptoms may be necessary, especially if they experience hallucinations, paranoia, and delusions, thus negatively impacting patient and caregiver safety and quality of life. According to the Beers Criteria (2019), when antipsychotic drugs are deemed necessary, Olanzapine and Quetiapine are recommended after risks are explained to caregivers and with ongoing risk assessments.

OTHER CONSIDERATIONS

- Abnormal antidiuretic hormone secretion (SIADH)
- Avoid the use of SGAs due to side effect risk of prolonging the QTc interval
- Fall risk
- FDA boxed warning of increased incidence of stroke in older adult patients with dementia
- Higher hospitalization rates
- Hyponatremia
- Increased rate of cognitive decline
- Increased mortality risk
- Psychotropic medications are associated with an increased risk for falls
- Start at low doses and titrate slowly

MEASURING AND MONITORING THERAPEUTIC RESPONSE

Currently, there are no universally accepted scales to measure recovery of schizophrenia; therefore, assessments are based on the diagnostic interview supplemented by collateral information. Achieving and maintaining remission is the primary aim of treatment. Remission refers to a period of time that is free of or has minimal symptoms that negatively impact behavior or functioning for at least 6 months (APA, 2013). Over the course of schizophrenia, psychotic symptoms can fluctuate, and clinician decision-making regarding treatment is influenced by individual response and side effects, as well as the phase of illness (acute vs. stable; Remington et al., 2017).

KEY POINTS

- Set realistic goals.
- Provide options of oral or depot medication formulations (Remington et al., 2017).
- After resolution of positive symptoms from the first episode of schizophrenia, duration of antipsychotic therapy use should be no less than 12 to 18 months (Begemann et al., 2020; Remington et al., 2017).
- After resolution of positive symptoms from subsequent acute episodes of schizophrenia, antipsychotic medication should be offered for 2 to 5 years (Remington et al., 2017).
- After medication adjustments (up or down), medication should be continued for at least 4 weeks unless intolerant to medication.
- After a 4-week follow-up assessment, partial responses should be reassessed in 8 weeks unless intolerant to medication.

WHEN TO REFER

- Psychotic episodes
- Agitation or extremely bothered by hallucinations
- Extreme mood or personality changes
- Severe medication side effects
- Risk of suicide or hurting themselves or others
- Symptom control has not been attainable as outpatient

SUMMARY

Although symptoms of schizophrenia vary in severity over time, individuals with schizophrenia require lifelong treatment. Individuals with schizophrenia often lack awareness that their difficulties can result in problems that affect many areas of life. Assertive community treatment (ACT) is a multidisciplinary team approach to intensive case management for community mental health services that has been developed for individuals with serious mental illness to provide support, education, and guidance to patients and caregivers. These programs incorporate clinical services, community outreach, and holistic approaches to reduce hospitalization rates and help with disease management. Services include medication management, housing, finances, rehabilitation, social services, and assistance in routine practical skills such as shopping and use of public transportation (Bond & Drake, 2015). Early, patient-centered treatment and management help to reduce symptoms before serious complications arise and patient and family psychoeducation help improve patient's quality of life and well-being.

Table 7.5

First-Generation Antipsychotic Agents

Generic Name (Brand Name)	Dosage Forms	FDA Approval	Clinical Considerations
Chlorpromazine (Thorazine)	Tablets Injectable Solution	*Adults:* schizophrenia, nausea/vomiting, preoperative apprehension, intraoperative sedation, intractable hiccups, acute intermittent porphyria *Off-Label:* migraine headache *Pediatrics:* behavioral disorders/hyperactivity, nausea/vomiting, preoperative apprehension (6 years and older) *Older Adult Considerations:* *,**	FDA black-box warnings for prolonged QTc-interval—monitor cardiac function. Monitor side effects: EPS, tachycardia, agranulocytosis, aplastic anemia, neuroleptic malignant syndrome, thermo-dysregulation, TD, akathisia, sedation, parkinsonism.
Fluphenazine (Prolixin)	Tablet Liquid Acute IM Depot IM	*Adults:* schizophrenia *Non-FDA:* Tourette syndrome, chorea, dementia, agitation *Pediatrics:* safety in pediatric use has not been established *Older Adult Considerations:* Start at 1–2.5 mg per day and increase gradually. *,**	Conversion from PO to the IM dose: 1.25 times the PO dose IM every 2 to 4 weeks. Monitor cardiac function. Metabolized primarily in the liver. Monitor side effects: EPS, tachycardia, priapism, torsades de pointes, agranulocytosis, aplastic anemia, neuroleptic malignant syndrome, thermo-dysregulation, TD, akathisia, sedation, parkinsonism.
Haloperidol (Haldol)	Tablet Liquid Acute IM Depot IM	*Adults:* schizophrenia, Tourette syndrome *Non-FDA:* severe anorexia nervosa, OCD, PTSD, nausea, severe anxiety, agitation *Off-Label:* IV use	Conversion: 20 times the oral daily dose (mg/day) X 1 month, divided into two biweekly injections. Monitor cardiac function. Metabolized primarily in the liver.

*Start at the lowest dosage and titrate slowly while monitoring the patient for any side effects.
**Avoid for behavior issues (dementia or delirium) in older adults due to increased risk of cerebrovascular accident and mortality. Avoid in older adults with history of falls and/or fractures due to potent anticholinergic and sedative effects unless no other safer alternative is available. Avoid use in older patients with Parkinson's disease since dopamine-receptor antagonists may worsen parkinsonian symptoms (Beers Criteria, 2019).

(*continued*)

Table 7.5

First-Generation Antipsychotic Agents (*continued*)

Generic Name (Brand Name)	Dosage Forms	FDA Approval	Clinical Considerations
		Pediatrics: schizophrenia (3 years and over), Tourette disorder (3 years and over), behavioral disorders (3 years and over), acute agitation (12 years and over) *Older Adult Considerations:* Start with 0.5 mg once or twice per day. *,**	Monitor side effects: EPS, tachycardia, priapism, torsades de pointes, agranulocytosis, aplastic anemia, neuroleptic malignant syndrome, thermo-dysregulation, TD, akathisia, sedation, parkinsonism.
Loxapine (Loxitane Adasuve)	Tablets Aerosol Powder Breath Activated, Inhalation	*Adults:* schizophrenia, schizoaffective disorder, bipolar I disorder, drug-induced psychosis *Non-FDA:* psychosis, agitation *Pediatrics:* safety in pediatric use has not been established. *Older Adult Considerations:* *,**	Adasuve administered only by a healthcare professional-Pulmonary assessment before and after. Instructions for use: Patient exhales fully, uses inhaler on inspiration and holds breath at least 10 seconds. Discard after one use.
Perphenazine (Trilafon)	Tablets IM injection	*Adults:* schizophrenia, nausea/vomiting *Off-Label:* intractable hiccups *Pediatrics:* safety in pediatric use has not been established under the age of 12; approved for use in patients with schizophrenia *Off-Label:* intractable hiccups *Older Adult Considerations:* *,**	*Monitor Cardiac Function:* Monitor side effects: EPS, tachycardia, priapism, torsades de pointes, agranulocytosis, aplastic anemia, neuroleptic malignant syndrome, thermo-dysregulation, TD, akathisia, sedation.
Pimozide (Orap)	Tablets	*Adults:* Tourette disorder *Non-FDA:* delusional parasitosis, schizophrenia *Pediatrics:* Tourette disorder *Off-Label:* schizophrenia *Older Adult Considerations:* ***	For doses over 4 mg per day in adults, CYP2D6 genotyping is required. For doses over 0.05 mg/kg per day in children, GYP2D genotyping is required. Discontinue gradually to avoid any symptoms of withdrawal.

*Start at the lowest dosage and titrate slowly while monitoring the patient for any side effects.
**Avoid for behavior issues (dementia or delirium) in older adults due to increased risk of cerebrovascular accident and mortality. Avoid in older adults with history of falls and/or fractures due to potent anticholinergic and sedative effects unless no other safer alternative is available. Avoid use in older patients with Parkinson's disease since dopamine-receptor antagonists may worsen parkinsonian symptoms (Beers Criteria, 2019).

(*continued*)

Table 7.5

First-Generation Antipsychotic Agents (*continued*)

Generic Name (Brand Name)	Dosage Forms	FDA Approval	Clinical Considerations
Thioridazine (Mellaril)	Tablets	*Adults:* schizophrenia *Pediatrics:* schizophrenia *Older Adult Considerations:* *,**	Individuals who do not respond adequately to other antipsychotic drugs; failed response refers to at least two trials, each with a different antipsychotic drug profile, at an adequate dose and for adequate duration.
Thiothixene (Navane)	Capsules	*Adults:* schizophrenia *Pediatrics:* safety in pediatric use has not been established under the age of 12, schizophrenia *Older Adult Considerations:* *,**	Monitor side effects: EPS, tachycardia, priapism, torsades de pointes, agranulocytosis, aplastic anemia, neuroleptic malignant syndrome, thermo-dysregulation, TD, akathisia, sedation, parkinsonism.
Trifluoperazine (Stelazine)	Tablets	*Adults:* schizophrenia, anxiety *Pediatrics:* schizophrenia *Older Adult Considerations:* *,**	Avoid use of venlafaxine due to increased risk of neuroleptic malignant syndrome and increased cardiac risks.

*Start at the lowest dosage and titrate slowly while monitoring the patient for any side effects.
**Avoid for behavior issues (dementia or delirium) in older adults due to increased risk of cerebrovascular accident and mortality. Avoid in older adults with history of falls and/or fractures due to potent anticholinergic and sedative effects unless no other safer alternative is available. Avoid use in older patients with Parkinson's disease since dopamine-receptor antagonists may worsen parkinsonian symptoms (Beers Criteria, 2019).
EPS, extrapyramidal symptoms; FDA, U.S. Food and Drug Administration; GAD, general anxiety disorder; IM, intramuscularly; IV, intravenously; MDD, major depressive disorder; OCD, obsessive-compulsive disorder; ODT, orally disintegrating tablet; PO, by mouth; PTSD, posttraumatic stress disorder; TD, tardive dyskinesia.

RESOURCES

- American Psychiatric Association (APA): Practice guideline for the treatment of patients with schizophrenia, third edition https://s21151.pcdn.co/wp-content/uploads/APA-Practice-Guideline-for-the-Treatment-of-Patients-with-Schizophrenia-3rd-Edition-SRC-1-8-21-CMMC-1.pdf
- American College of Radiology (ACR): ACR Appropriateness Criteria on acute mental status change, delirium, and new onset psychosis https://pubmed.ncbi.nlm.nih.gov/31054753

Table 7.6

Second-Generation Antipsychotic Agents

Generic Name (Brand Name)	Dosage Forms	FDA Approval	Clinical Considerations
Aripiprazole (Abilify, Abilify Maintena; Depot Aristada Inito-aripiprazole lauroxil, Abilify MyCite; Maintenance Kit Abilify MyCite Starter Kit)	Tablets ODT Liquid IM Acute IM Depot IM (Abilify Maintena) Single-Dose Injection Aristada Initio (Aripiprazole Lauroxil)	*Adults:* schizophrenia, bipolar disorder, MDD *Non-FDA Uses:* borderline personality disorder *Pediatrics:* schizophrenia (13 years and older), bipolar disorder (10 years and older), autism disorder (6 years and older) *Older Adult Considerations:* Follow standard adult dosing*,**	*,***Conservative doses are recommended when used with potent CYP2D6 and/or 3A4 inhibitors. If naïve to aripiprazole, establish tolerability with oral aripiprazole prior to treatment with Aristada Initio, Aristada. All doses of Aristada may be administered in the gluteal or deltoid muscle (441 mg dose only). Avoid injecting both Aristada Initio and Aristada concomitantly into the same deltoid or gluteal muscle. Dosage adjustments for Aristada Initio are not available—it is supplied in a single-dose prefilled syringe.
Asenapine (Saphris)	Tablets (Sublingual)	*Adults:* schizophrenia, bipolar I disorder *Non-FDA:* dementia, substance abuse, anorexia nervosa, OCD, PTSD, GAD, Tourette syndrome, MDD, borderline personality disorder, Parkinson disease, hiccups, nausea/vomiting, delirium *Pediatrics:* bipolar I disorder (10 to 17 years of age) *Older Adult Considerations:* *,**,***	Instruct patient to avoid eating or drinking 10 minutes after each dose, and to not chew, cut, crush, or swallow the tablet whole due to ↓ gastrointestinal absorption; rather, let it dissolve under the tongue. Can be prescribed PRN for mania and agitation, due to rapid onset of action.

*Start at the lowest dosage and titrate slowly while monitoring the patient for any side effects.
**Avoid for behavior issues (dementia or delirium) in older adults due to increased risk of cerebrovascular accident and mortality. Avoid in older adults with history of falls and/or fractures due to potent anticholinergic and sedative effects unless no other safer alternative is available. Avoid use in older patients with Parkinson's disease since dopamine-receptor antagonists may worsen parkinsonian symptoms (Beers Criteria, 2019).
***Discontinue if absolute neutrophil count (ANC) falls below 1,000 and/or white blood cells (WBC) decrease for unknown reason. Severe neutropenia (ANC < 1,000/mm^3): Discontinue treatment.

(*continued*)

Table 7.6

Second-Generation Antipsychotic Agents (*continued*)

Generic Name (Brand Name)	Dosage Forms	FDA Approval	Clinical Considerations
Brexpiprazole (Rexulti)	Tablets	*Adults:* schizophrenia, adjunct for treatment-resistant depression *Pediatrics:* safety in pediatric use has not been established *Older Adult Considerations:* *,**,*** Patients with dementia-related psychosis may be at higher risk of death.	Depression: May be increased in weekly intervals up to 1 mg once daily and then up to 2 mg once daily. Do not exceed 3 mg per day.
Cariprazine (Vraylar)	Capsules	*Adults:* schizophrenia, bipolar I disorder, acute mania *Pediatrics:* safety in pediatric use has not been established. *Older Adult Considerations:* *,**,***	Drug has a long half-life.
Clozapine (Clozaril) {see monitoring and special considerations section on clozapine}	Tablets ODT Liquid	*Adults:* schizophrenia (treatment resistant) *Non-FDA Uses:* dementia, substance abuse, anorexia nervosa, OCD, PTSD, GAD, Tourette syndrome, MDD, borderline personality disorder, Parkinson's disease, hiccups, nausea/vomiting, delirium *Pediatrics:* safety in pediatric use has not been established *Older Adult Considerations:* Start with lowest dosage; may be increased more slowly than in younger adults *,**,***	Must obtain CBC count that shows ANC count over 2,000 mm^3 and WBC count over 3,500 mm^3 before initiating.*** Has shown to be effective in recurrent suicidal behavior for individuals with schizophrenia or schizoaffective disorder.

*Start at the lowest dosage and titrate slowly while monitoring the patient for any side effects.
**Avoid for behavior issues (dementia or delirium) in older adults due to increased risk of cerebrovascular accident and mortality. Avoid in older adults with history of falls and/or fractures due to potent anticholinergic and sedative effects unless no other safer alternative is available. Avoid use in older patients with Parkinson's disease since dopamine-receptor antagonists may worsen parkinsonian symptoms (Beers Criteria, 2019).
***Discontinue if absolute neutrophil count (ANC) falls below 1,000 and/or white blood cells (WBC) decrease for unknown reason. Severe neutropenia (ANC < 1,000/mm^3): Discontinue treatment.

(*continued*)

Table 7.6

Second-Generation Antipsychotic Agents (*continued*)

Generic Name (Brand Name)	Dosage Forms	FDA Approval	Clinical Considerations
Iloperidone (Fanapt)	Tablets	*Adults:* schizophrenia *Pediatrics:* safety in pediatric use has not been established *Older Adult Considerations:* follow standard adult dosing *,**,***	Monitor BP.
Lumateperone (Caplyta)	Tablets	*Adults:* schizophrenia *Pediatrics:* safety in pediatric use has not been established *Older Adult Considerations:* patients with dementia-related psychosis are at increased risk of life-threatening events *,**,***	Take at night to avoid sedation. Monitor BP.
Lurasidone (Latuda)	Tablets	*Adults:* schizophrenia, bipolar depression *Pediatrics:* safety in pediatric use has not been established *Older Adult Considerations:* *, **, ***	Take with food > 350 calories.
Olanzapine (Zyprexa, Olanzapine-fluoxetine combination [Symbyax])	Tablet ODT Acute IM Depot IM Olanzapine-Fluoxetine Capsule	*Adults:* schizophrenia, bipolar mania, agitation, bipolar depression *Off-Label:* MDD, nausea/vomiting *Pediatrics:* bipolar I disorder (13 year and over), schizophrenia (13 years and over), bipolar disorder (10 years and over) *Off-Label:* stuttering (over 12 years), start with lowest dose *Older Adult Considerations:* start with lowest dosage *, **, ***	May be adjusted in patients who smoke.

*Start at the lowest dosage and titrate slowly while monitoring the patient for any side effects.
**Avoid for behavior issues (dementia or delirium) in older adults due to increased risk of cerebrovascular accident and mortality. Avoid in older adults with history of falls and/or fractures due to potent anticholinergic and sedative effects unless no other safer alternative is available. Avoid use in older patients with Parkinson's disease since dopamine-receptor antagonists may worsen parkinsonian symptoms (Beers Criteria, 2019).
***Discontinue if absolute neutrophil count (ANC) falls below 1,000 and/or white blood cells (WBC) decrease for unknown reason. Severe neutropenia (ANC < 1,000/mm^3): Discontinue treatment.

(*continued*)

Table 7.6

Second-Generation Antipsychotic Agents (*continued*)

Generic Name (Brand Name)	Dosage Forms	FDA Approval	Clinical Considerations
Paliperidone (Invega, Invega Sustenna; Invega Trinza)	ER Tablets Monthly Depot IM (Invega Sustenna)	*Adults:* schizophrenia, schizoaffective disorder *Non-FDA Uses:* bipolar I disorder *Pediatrics:* safety in pediatric use has not been established under the age of 12 (ER tablets only); schizophrenia *Older Adult Considerations:* follow standard adult dosing *, **, ***	Advise patients to swallow tablets whole. Do not break or chew. Establish tolerability by using at least 2 PO doses before administering. Administered in the deltoid muscle.
Quetiapine (Seroquel, Seroquel XR)	IR Tablet ER Tablet	*Adults:* schizophrenia, bipolar mania, adjunct to antidepressant MDD, agitation *Off-Label:* alcohol dependence, insomnia *Pediatrics:* schizophrenia (12 years and older), bipolar I disorder mania (10 years and older) *Older Adult Considerations:* *, **, ***	Approved for adjunctive treatment of MDD
Risperidone (Risperdal, Perseris; Risperdal Consta)	Tablets Oral Solution ODT Depot IM	*Adults:* schizophrenia, bipolar mania, bipolar disorder *Off-Label:* Tourette syndrome, PTSD *Pediatrics:* schizophrenia (13 years and older), bipolar mania (10 years and older), irritability associated with autistic disorder (5 years and older) *Depot IM:* safety in pediatric use has not been established *Older Adult Considerations:* *, **, ***	Ensure tolerance of oral tablets before administering IM forms.

*Start at the lowest dosage and titrate slowly while monitoring the patient for any side effects.
**Avoid for behavior issues (dementia or delirium) in older adults due to increased risk of cerebrovascular accident and mortality. Avoid in older adults with history of falls and/or fractures due to potent anticholinergic and sedative effects unless no other safer alternative is available. Avoid use in older patients with Parkinson's disease since dopamine-receptor antagonists may worsen parkinsonian symptoms (Beers Criteria, 2019).
***Discontinue if absolute neutrophil count (ANC) falls below 1,000 and/or white blood cells (WBC) decrease for unknown reason. Severe neutropenia (ANC < 1,000/mm^3): Discontinue treatment.

(*continued*)

Table 7.6

Second-Generation Antipsychotic Agents (*continued*)

Generic Name (Brand Name)	Dosage Forms	FDA Approval	Clinical Considerations
Ziprasidone (Geodon)	Capsules Acute IM	*Adults:* schizophrenia, bipolar I disorder, postponing relapse in schizophrenia, acute agitation in schizophrenia (IM), acute mania/mixed mania, bipolar maintenance *Non-FDA Uses:* schizoaffective disorder *Pediatrics:* safety in pediatric use has not been established *Off-Label:* Tourette syndrome *Older Adult Considerations:* follow standard adult dosing**	Monitor cardiac function. Take with food to increase bioavailability.
Pimavanserin (Nuplazid)	Capsule Tablets	*Adults:* hallucinations and delusions associated with Parkinson's disease psychosis *Pediatrics:* safety in pediatric use has not been established	No titration is used; focus on once a day dosing.

*Start at the lowest dosage and titrate slowly while monitoring the patient for any side effects.
**Avoid for behavior issues (dementia or delirium) in older adults due to increased risk of cerebrovascular accident and mortality. Avoid in older adults with history of falls and/or fractures due to potent anticholinergic and sedative effects unless no other safer alternative is available. Avoid use in older patients with Parkinson's disease since dopamine-receptor antagonists may worsen parkinsonian symptoms (Beers Criteria, 2019).
***Discontinue if absolute neutrophil count (ANC) falls below 1,000 and/or white blood cells (WBC) decrease for unknown reason. Severe neutropenia (ANC < 1,000/mm^3): Discontinue treatment.
BP, blood pressure; CBC, complete blood count; FDA, U.S. Food and Drug Administration; GAD, general anxiety disorder; IM, intramuscularly; MDD, major depressive disorder; OCD, obsessive-compulsive disorder; ODT, orally disintegrating tablet; PTSD, posttraumatic stress disorder

- APA: Practice guideline on the use of antipsychotics to treat agitation or psychosis in patients with dementia https://psychiatryonline.org/doi/pdf/10.1176/appi.books.9780890426807
- American Academy of Child and Adolescent Psychiatry (AACAP): Practice parameter for the assessment and treatment of children and adolescents with schizophrenia https://www.jaacap.org/article/S0890-8567(13)00112-3/fulltext
- Choosing Wisely: Don't prescribe antipsychotic medications to patients for any indication without appropriate initial evaluation and appropriate ongoing monitoring

- Choosing Wisely: Don't routinely prescribe two or more antipsychotic medications concurrently
- NICE: Clinical guideline on psychosis and schizophrenia in children and young people—Recognition and management https://www.nice.org.uk/guidance/cg155
- NICE: Quality standard on bipolar disorder, psychosis, and schizophrenia in children and young people https://www.nice.org.uk/guidance/qs80
- NICE: Quality standard on psychosis and schizophrenia in adults
- NICE: Clinical guideline on psychosis and schizophrenia in adults—Prevention and management https://www.nice.org.uk/guidance/cg178

REVIEW QUESTIONS

1. To begin administering Clozaril, a minimum absolute neutrophil count (ANC) value at baseline of _______ is required for the general population and a minimum of _____for individuals with benign ethnic neutropenia.
   a. 1,500/uL, 1,000/uL
   b. 1,000/uL, 500/uL
   c. 500/uL, 500/uL
   d. 1,000/uL, 1,500/uL
2. Which one of the following statements best describes the rationale for avoiding antipsychotic medication use in older adults?
   a. According to the Beers Criteria, antipsychotics have been identified as potentially inappropriate medications and are to be avoided in patients 65 years and older but are safe to use for insomnia since they do promote sleep.
   b. SGAs increase the risk of cerebrovascular accidents (stroke), slow the rate of cognitive decline, and slow mortality in older adults with dementia.
   c. Antipsychotics should be used with caution in older adults due to their potential to trigger inappropriate antidiuretic hormone secretion (SIADH), cause hyponatremia, increase stroke risk, increase rate of cognitive decline, and increase mortality.
   d. Antipsychotics would not help restore memory in older adults.
3. The main difference between SGAs or atypical antipsychotics and FGAs or typical antipsychotics is that SGAs have which one of the following?
   a. Dopaminergic and serotonergic blocking properties
   b. Serotonergic blocking properties and dopamine agonist properties
   c. Dopaminergic and serotonergic agonist properties
   d. Neither dopaminergic nor serotonergic blocking properties
4. Tongue protrusion, side-to-side movement of the jaw, lip smacking, puckering and pursing, rapid eye blinking, and movements of the arms, legs, and trunk are signs of a neurologic disorder associated with antipsychotic medications that is referred to as ___________________________.
   a. Akinesia
   b. Tardive dyskinesia

c. Cholinergic antagonism
d. Dystonia

5. Treatment for extrapyramidal symptoms (EPS) includes all of the following except for which one?
   a. Prescribe benztropine (Cogentin).
   b. Lower medication dosage.
   c. Stop and change medication.
   d. Prescribe dantrolene.

REFERENCES

Abou-Setta, A. M., Mousavi, S. S., Spooner, C., Schouten, J. R., Pasichnyk, D., Armijo-Olivo, S., Beauith, A., Seida, J. C., Dursun, S., Newton, A. S., & Hartling, L. (2012). *First-generation versus second-generation antipsychotics in adults: Comparative effectiveness (Comparative Effectiveness Review No. 63).* Agency for Healthcare Research and Quality. https://www.ncbi.nlm.nih.gov/books/NBK107254/pdf/Bookshelf_NBK107254.pdf

Addington, D., Abidi, S., Garcia-Ortega, I., Honer, W. G., & Ismail, Z. (2017). Canadian guidelines for the assessment and diagnosis of patients with schizophrenia spectrum and other psychotic disorders. *Canadian Journal of Psychiatry, 62*(9), 594–603. https://doi.org/10.1177/0706743717719899

American Geriatrics Society Beers Criteria® Update Expert Panel (2019). American Geriatrics Society 2019 Updated AGS Beers Criteria® for Potentially Inappropriate Medication Use in Older Adults. *Journal of the American Geriatrics Society, 67*(4), 674–694. https://doi.org/10.1111/jgs.15767

American Psychiatric Association. (2013). *Diagnostic and statistical manual of mental disorders* (5th ed.). https://doi.org/10.1176/appi.books.9780890425596

Begemann, M., Thompson, I. A., Veling, W., Gangadin, S. S., Geraets, C., van 't Hag, E., Müller-Kuperus, S. J., Oomen, P. P., Voppel, A. E., van der Gaag, M., Kikkert, M. J., Van Os, J., Smit, H., Knegtering, R. H., Wiersma, S., Stouten, L. H., Gijsman, H. J., Wunderink, L., Staring, A., ... Sommer, I. (2020). To continue or not to continue? Antipsychotic medication maintenance versus dose-reduction/discontinuation in first episode psychosis: HAMLETT, a pragmatic multicenter single-blind randomized controlled trial. *Trials, 21*(1), 147. https://doi.org/10.1186/s13063-019-3822-5

Berman, B. D. (2011). Neuroleptic malignant syndrome: A review for neurohospitalists. *The Neurohospitalist, 1*(1), 41–47. https://doi.org/10.1177/1941875210386491

Bond, G. R., & Drake, R. E. (2015). The critical ingredients of assertive community treatment. *World Psychiatry, 14*(2), 240–242. https://doi.org/10.1002/wps.20234

Calabrese, J., & Al Khalili, Y. (n.d.). *Psychosis.* StatPearls. Retrieved July 17, 2021, from https://www.ncbi.nlm.nih.gov/books/NBK546579

Clozapine Risk Evaluation and Mitigation Strategy . (n.d.). *Homepage.* Retrieved July 17, 2021, from https://www.clozapinerems.com

Fatemi, S. H., & Folsom, T. D. (2009). The neurodevelopmental hypothesis of schizophrenia, revisited. *Schizophrenia Bulletin, 35*(3), 528–548. https://doi.org/10.1093/schbul/sbn187

Hany, M., Rehman, B., Azhar, Y., & Chapman, J. (n.d.). *Schizophrenia.* StatPearls. Retrieved July 17, 2021, from https://www.ncbi.nlm.nih.gov/books/NBK539864

Hasan, A., Falkai, P., Wobrock, T., Lieberman, J., Glenthoj, B., Gattaz, W. F., Thibaut, F., Möller, H. J., & World Federation of Societies of Biological Psychiatry Task

Force on Treatment Guidelines for Schizophrenia. (2012). World Federation of Societies of Biological Psychiatry (WFSBP) guidelines for biological treatment of schizophrenia, part 1: Update 2012 on the acute treatment of schizophrenia and the management of treatment resistance. *World Journal of Biological Psychiatry, 13*(5), 318–378. https://doi.org/10.3109/15622975.2012.696143

Health Quality Ontario. (2018). Cognitive behavioral therapy for psychosis: A health technology assessment. *Ontario Health Technology Assessment Series, 18*(5), 1–141. https://www.ncbi.nlm.nih.gov/pmc/articles/PMC6235075

Koran, L. M., Hanna, G. L., Hollander, E., Nestadt, G., Simpson, H. B., & American Psychiatric Association. Practice guideline for the treatment of patients with obsessive-compulsive disorder. Arlington, VA: American Psychiatric Association, 2007. Available online at http//www.psych.org/psych_pract/treatg/pg/prac_ guide .cfm. *The American Journal of Psychiatry, 164*(7 Suppl), 5–53.

Meltzer, H. Y., Alphs, L., Green, A. I., Altamura, A. C., Anand, R., Bertoldi, A., Bourgeois, M., Chouinard, G., Islam, M. Z., Kane, J., Krishnan, R., Lindenmayer, J. P., Potkin, S., & International Suicide Prevention Trial Study Group. (2003). Clozapine treatment for suicidality in schizophrenia: International Suicide Prevention Trial (InterSePT). *Archives of General Psychiatry, 60*(1), 82–91. https://doi.org/10.1001/archpsyc.60.1.82

Merrill, A. M., Karcher, N. R., Cicero, D. C., Becker, T. M., Docherty, A. R., & Kerns, J. G. (2017). Evidence that communication impairment in schizophrenia is associated with generalized poor task performance. *Psychiatry Research, 249*, 172–179. https://doi.org/10.1016/j.psychres.2016.12.051

National Institute for Health and Care Excellence. (2013). *Psychosis and schizophrenia in children and young people: Recognition and management.* https://www.nice.org.uk/guidance/cg155/resources/psychosis-and-schizophrenia-in-children-and-young-people-recognition-and-management-pdf-35109632980933

National Institute for Health and Care Excellence. (2015). *Psychosis and schizophrenia in children and young people: Evidence.* https://www.ncbi.nlm.nih.gov/books/NBK552055/pdf/Bookshelf_NBK552055.pdf

Ortiz-Orendain, J., Castiello-de Obeso, S., Colunga-Lozano, L. E., Hu, Y., Maayan, N., & Adams, C. E. (2017). Antipsychotic combinations for schizophrenia. *The Cochrane Database of Systematic Reviews, 6*(6), Article CD009005. https://doi.org/10.1002/14651858.CD009005.pub2

Pillay, J., Boylan, K., Carrey, N., Newton, A., Vandermeer, B., Nuspl, M., MacGregor, R., Jafri, S. H. A., Featherston, R., & Hartling, L. (2017). *First- and second-generation antipsychotics in children and young adults: Systematic review update (Comparative Effectiveness Review No. 184).* Agency for Healthcare Research and Quality. https://www.ncbi.nlm.nih.gov/books/NBK442352/pdf/Bookshelf_NBK442352.pdf

Remington, G., Addington, D., Honer, W., Ismail, Z., Raedler, T., & Teehan, M. (2017). Guidelines for the pharmacotherapy of schizophrenia in adults. *Canadian Journal of Psychiatry, 62*(9), 604–616. https://doi.org/10.1177/0706743717720448

Sheffield, J. M., Karcher, N. R., & Barch, D. M. (2018). Cognitive deficits in psychotic disorders: A lifespan perspective. *Neuropsychology Review, 28*(4), 509–533. https://doi.org/10.1007/s11065-018-9388-2

The 2019 American Geriatrics Society Beers Criteria Update Expert Panel. (2019). American Geriatrics Society 2019 updated AGS Beers Criteria for potentially inappropriate medication use in older adults. *Journal of the American Geriatrics Society, 67*(4), 674–694. https://doi.org/10.1111/jgs.15767

8

Mood Stabilizers

Bipolar disorder (BD) is a serious chronic disorder associated with high morbidity and mortality rates. BD is a type of mental disorder characterized by cycles of fluctuating energy and mood swings that range from elation and/or grandiosity, excitement, and explosiveness to irritability and low or depressed moods that are associated with changes in sleep. Mood features are accompanied by episodes of mania, hypomania, mixed manic-depressive states, psychosis, intense anxiety, and prominent major depression symptoms, all of which can lead to potentially severe functional impairment (Hui Poon et al., 2015). Substance abuse, high rates of suicide, accidents, cognitive deficits, increased mortality rates from co-occurring medical and psychiatric illnesses, high disability rates, high relapse rates, high social and economic costs, and reduced quality of life are linked to BD despite significant advances in understanding the underlying neurobiology of BD and availability of pharmacologic and psychotherapy treatment options (Hui Poon et al., 2015; Maletic & Raison, 2014). Individuals with bipolar and related disorders are also more likely to experience concurrent anxiety, panic, elevated levels of suicidality (10 to 30 times higher than that of the general population), employment instability, and difficulties with interpersonal relationships (Dome et al., 2019; Ferrari et al., 2016). According to Dome et al. (2019), 4% to 19% of individuals with BD die by suicide, and 20% to 60% attempt suicide during their lifetime.

In this chapter you will learn:

1. How to interpret specific manifestations of bipolar and related mood disorders
2. How to compare pharmacologic options for bipolar and related disorders

3. How to name five key features of bipolar and related disorders
4. How to identify screening tools for bipolar disorders
5. How to utilize medication safety considerations in prescribing and managing bipolar and related disorders
6. How to assess therapeutic responses in bipolar and related disorders

Essential Facts

- Major depressive features and mixed states carry the highest risk of suicide, whereas suicidal behavior is rarely present in (euphoric) mania, hypomania, and euthymic periods.
- Based on clinical history, previous suicide attempts are considered to be one of the most powerful single predictors of future attempts and suicide death risk.

BD is associated with high levels of psychologic stressors that burden patients, families, and society. Individuals with BD have poor life expectancies with an estimated decreased life span of approximately 9 to 17 years compared with the general population (Dome et al., 2019; Ferrari et al., 2016).

This chapter will provide an overview of mood disorders, including bipolar I (BP-I), bipolar II (BP-II), cyclothymia disorder (cyclothymic disorder), substance/medication-induced bipolar and related disorder, bipolar and related disorder due to another medical condition, and other specified bipolar and related disorders, as well as highlight the key features and evidence in assessing, diagnosing, treating, and managing these disorders across the life span.

Essential Facts

The peak onset of BD is 15 to 19 years of age.

DIAGNOSTIC CRITERIA FOR BIPOLAR I DISORDER

The primary clinical symptoms of BD are a pattern of recurrent manic, depressive, and mixed features that may or may not be associated with precipitating events or stressors. The expression of mood disturbance may present as (a) bipolar (mania and depression), (b) unipolar (mania only), and (c) mixed (co-occurring mania and depression; see Table 8.1). According to the *Diagnostic and Statistical Manual of Mental Disorders* (5th ed.; *DSM-5*; American Psychiatric Association [APA], 2013), the criterion for BP-I requires at least one manic episode lasting a minimum of 1 weeks' duration (must be present most of the day, nearly every day, or any duration of time if patient is hospitalized) that includes at least four symptoms of mania (i.e., inflated self-esteem, disinhibition, pressured speech, decreased need for sleep). If the individual's mood presents as irritable, three symptoms of mania are required for diagnosis. For example, increased energy, excessive optimism, and flight of ideas must be present and cause social and/or occupational impairment that cannot be better explained by schizophrenia, another mental health disorder, general medical condition, medication (except antidepressant or electroconvulsive therapy [ECT]), or other symptoms induced by a substance.

Table 8.1

Symptoms of Mania, Hypomania, Depressive, and Mixed Features

Manic features	■ Observable increase in energy (mania or hypomania) ■ Expansive mood ■ Increase in activity ■ Decreased need for sleep ■ Frequently distracted ■ Impulsive behaviors ■ Easily distracted ■ Abnormal and persistent goal-directed behaviors (socially, occupational, in school, or sexually) ■ Psychomotor agitation (purposeless nongoal-directed activity). ■ Sexually risky or occupationally risky behavior (shopping sprees, gambling, sexual indiscretions) ■ Inflated self-esteem ■ Unrealistic beliefs of grandeur ■ Rapid speech and talkative ■ Flight of ideas ■ Observable and/or subjective mood elevation with functional impairment(s)
Hypomania features	■ Inflated self-esteem ■ Flight of ideas ■ Easily distracted ■ Decreased need for sleep ■ Increase in risky behavior (shopping sprees, gambling, sexual indiscretions) ■ Increased goal-directed activities ■ Observable changes in mood to abnormally and persistently elevated, expansive, energetic, or irritable mood (not as extreme as mania with less functional impairment) ■ Differs from mania by the intensity and duration of mood symptoms ■ Features are required to persist for at least 4 days (mania requires at least 7 days) to meet diagnostic criteria ■ May mildly impair or improve an individual's psychosocial and occupational functioning ■ Absence of psychosis ■ Does not require hospitalization

(*continued*)

Table 8.1

Symptoms of Mania, Hypomania, Depressive, and Mixed Features (*continued*)

Major depressive features (see Chapter 5)	A minimum of at least five of the following symptoms for at least 2 weeks; at least one of the symptoms must be either dysphoria or anhedonia: ▪ Dysphoric or depressed mood most of the day, almost every day ▪ Anhedonia (diminished interest or pleasure in daily activities), most of the day, almost every day ▪ Weight changes (loss or weight gain) ▪ Change in appetite ▪ Insomnia or hypersomnia ▪ Psychomotor agitation ▪ Fatigue ▪ Thoughts of worthlessness ▪ Guilt ▪ Cognitive changes ▪ Suicidal ideation or suicide attempt
Mixed affective features	▪ Co-occurring symptoms of major depression, mania, and hypomania (feelings of extreme sadness, guilt, and worthlessness, while at the same time experiencing high energy and racing thoughts and speech)

DIAGNOSTIC CRITERIA FOR BIPOLAR II DISORDER

Hypomania is described as a period of observable elevated mood, disinhibition, increased self-esteem, and a decreased need for sleep. Individuals experiencing hypomania exhibit heightened energy and activity, euphoria, and elated states or irritability that lasts at least 4 consecutive days for most of the day without any significant functional impairments or need for hospitalization (APA, 2013; Goodwin et al., 2016). Criterion for BP-II diagnosis include no evidence of prior manic features, at least one or more past or present depressive features, and one or more hypomanic features. To meet criteria for a hypomanic feature, the individual's symptoms must include at least three or more hypomanic symptoms (see Table 8.1). If the individual demonstrates irritability, the individual must exhibit four or more symptoms that cannot be better explained by schizophrenia, another mental health disorder, general medical condition, medication (except antidepressant or ECT), or another substance. According to the *DSM-5* (APA, 2013), if hypomanic symptoms present following antidepressant use, symptoms of a full hypomanic episode must persist beyond the physiological effect of treatment is required for adequate diagnosis. Additionally, caution should be used when considering the diagnosis of BP-II when symptoms such as edginess, irritability or agitation emerge following antidepressant treatment since they are not sufficient to meet criteria for diagnosis.

Essential Facts

BP-I Diagnostic Criteria:

- It includes one or more features of mania.
- Hypomania may occur but is not required for diagnosis.

(*continued*)

Essential Facts (*continued*)

- Rule out the possibility that the mood symptoms are due to schizophrenia, another mental health disorder, or a general medical condition, or induced by a substance.

BP-II Diagnostic Criteria:

- It includes one or more features of hypomania.
- It includes one or more features of major depression.
- No history of mania is noted.
- Rule out the possibility that the mood symptoms are due to schizophrenia, another mental health disorder, or a general medical condition, or induced by a substance.

DIAGNOSTIC CRITERIA FOR CYCLOTHYMIA

Cyclothymia is a subtype of BD characterized by chronic and reactive mood fluctuations involving low-grade depressive and hypomanic symptoms. Cyclothymia can be associated with moodiness, irritability, and anxious and impulsive behaviors (Van Meter & Youngstrom, 2012). Individuals diagnosed with cyclothymia react to positive and negative events (real or perceived) with disproportionally intense reactions and may display a wide range of emotions.

To meet criteria for the diagnosis of cyclothymic disorder, an adult must have experienced a 2-year (1 year for children and adolescents) duration of numerous hypomanic and depressive symptoms without ever meeting the criteria for mania, hypomania, or major depression. Mood symptoms must be persistent, and the individual cannot be symptom-free for intervals longer than 2 months during the initial 2-year (1 year for children and adolescents) time frame. Additionally, cyclothymia (a) is not associated with schizophrenia or other mental or general medical conditions, (b) is not induced by medication or substance use, and (c) interferes with psychosocial functional impairments (APA, 2013). Tables 8.1 through 8.3 list the key features associated with bipolar spectrum disorders.

Essential Facts

There is a 15% to 50% risk that individuals with cyclothymic disorder will later develop BP-I disorder or BP-II disorder (APA, 2013).

Essential Facts

Although there is no formal criterion for *normal cycling, rapid cycling* refers to individuals who experience four or more episodes of mania or depression during a twelve-month period.

Table 8.2

Key Features of Bipolar and Related Disorders

Disorder	Key Features
BP-I	Individual experiences one or more manic features. Although not required for diagnosis, most individuals experience at least one episode of major depression and/or hypomania that is not better explained by schizoaffective disorder, schizophrenia, or other psychotic conditions. Identifiers to describe course of illness: ▪ Rapid cycling ▪ A seasonal pattern ▪ Psychotic features ▪ Catatonia ▪ Anxious distress ▪ Mixed features ▪ Melancholic features ▪ Atypical features ▪ Peripartum onset
BP-II	No reported manic episodes with a history of at least one hypomanic episode and at least one major depressive episode that is not better explained by schizoaffective disorder, schizophrenia, or other psychotic conditions. Although not required, may also experience: ▪ Psychotic features ▪ Rapid cycling ▪ Catatonia ▪ Anxious distress ▪ Mixed features
Cyclothymia disorder	▪ Cycles of hypomanic mood symptoms occur that do not meet the full criteria for hypomania and periods of depressive symptoms that do not meet the criteria for a major depressive episode. ▪ Symptoms persist over 2 or more consecutive years, during which the individual is symptomatic at least half the time and is not symptom-free for more than 2 consecutive months. ▪ Mood symptoms cause significant distress or psychosocial impairment; however, they are not caused by substance use or a medical condition. ▪ Mood symptoms in cyclothymic disorder are not better explained by other specified or unspecified schizophrenia spectrum conditions.
Substance/medication-induced bipolar and related disorder	A mood disturbance (elevated or irritable mood) that may be accompanied by depressed mood or anhedonia that presents during or soon after using substances (cocaine, stimulants, etc.) that cause significant distress or impair psychosocial functioning. Exceptions include: ▪ It is the result of antidepressant medication. ▪ Mood disturbance leads to the onset of substance intoxication or withdrawal, or exposure to substance. ▪ Mood disturbance lasts for 1 month or longer after cessation of acute intoxication or withdrawal. ▪ A prior history of recurrent mood episodes is reported. ▪ Disturbance in mood appears only during a period of delirium.

(continued)

Table 8.2

Key Features of Bipolar and Related Disorders (*continued*)

Disorder	Key Features
Bipolar and related disorder due to another medical condition	■ Disturbance in mood or bipolar symptoms occurs that causes significant distress or impairment in psychosocial functioning but does not meet the full criteria for a specific BD. ■ Specify the reason that the presenting symptoms do not meet criteria for BD. Document findings that indicate that the disturbance is caused by another medical condition. ■ Onset of the mood symptoms occurs during the first month of the onset of the medical condition. ■ Results in significant distress or impairs psychosocial functioning.
Other specified bipolar and related disorders	■ Mood symptomatology occurs that does not meet the complete criteria for a specific BD. ■ The patient experiences significant distress or impaired psychosocial functioning. ■ Identify the reason for not meeting criteria (short-duration hypomanic syndromes [1 to 3 days], hypomanic episodes without prior major depressive episode, short-duration cyclothymia, etc.).
Unspecified bipolar and related disorder	■ Significant distress or impaired psychosocial functioning occurs due to mood disturbance. ■ Does not meet the complete criteria for a specific BD but does not identify the reason for not meeting diagnostic criteria.

BD, bipolar disorder; BP-I, bipolar I; BP-II, bipolar II

Table 8.3

Mania, Hypomania, Depressive, and Mixed Episodes

Symptoms of mania	■ Observable increase in energy (mania or hypomania) ■ Increase in activity ■ Insomnia ■ Frequently distracted ■ Impulsive behaviors ■ Risky behavior ■ Unrealistic beliefs of grandeur ■ Rapid speech ■ Flight of ideas: difficulty keeping up or changes topics or patterns of thinking frequently ■ Observable and/or subjective mood elevation with functional impairment (APA, 2013; Goodwin et al., 2016)
Hypomania	■ An elated state where the individual experiences an elevated mood and exhibits more energy than usual but is not out of control and does not experience any significant functional impairments. Hypomania can also be described as a less severe form of mania (APA, 2013; Goodwin et al., 2016).
Mixed affective episodes	■ Symptoms of depression and mania or hypomania that co-occur that are not severe enough to cause a change in overall function

Essential Facts

DIG FAST is a mnemonic commonly used to remember the symptoms of mania:

- **D**istractibility and easy frustration
- **I**rresponsibility and erratic uninhibited behavior
- **G**randiosity
- **F**light of ideas
- **A**ctivity increased with weight loss and increased libido
- **S**leep is decreased
- **T**alkativeness

RISK FACTORS FOR BIPOLAR AND RELATED DISORDERS

- Brain structure and circuitry abnormalities
- Comorbid anxiety disorders
- Drug or alcohol abuse
- Environmental factors (adverse childhood events, maltreatment, trauma)
- Evidence of hypothyroidism or hyperthyroidism
- Family history of first-degree relative with major depressive disorder (MDD) or BD
- High family conflict
- Lack of family support
- Periods of high stress

Essential Facts

Family history is the greatest risk factor for BD; therefore, clinicians need to ask depressed individuals about a family history of BD.

POOR PROGNASTIC FACTORS

- Baseline severity
- Comorbidities
- Earlier onset of first depressive episode (younger than 25 years old)
- High family conflict (divorced, unmarried, or single parents, or social isolation)
- Increased mood cycling
- Increased suicide risk
- Lack of social and family support
- Longer duration of untreated illness
- Poor metabolizer genotype
- Predominant depressive polarity and mixed states

- Previous suicide attempt(s)
- Psychotic features
- Rapid-cycling pattern
- Severity of depression
- Worse quality of life

FAVORABLE PROGNASTIC OUTCOMES

- Diet
- Exercise
- Familial support
- Family psychoeducation
- Skill building
- Therapeutic alliance with clinician(s)
- Treatment adherence to medication
- Treatment adherence to substance misuse recovery programs

COMPLICATIONS

- Drug and alcohol use
- Financial problems
- Legal problems
- Poor work or school performance
- Problems with interpersonal relationships
- Suicide or suicide attempts

DIFFERENTIAL DIAGNOSIS

- Attention deficit hyperactivity disorder (ADHD)
- Autism spectrum disorder
- Bipolar or related disorder due to another medical condition
- Conduct disorder
- Cyclothymic disorder
- Disruptive mood dysregulation disorder
- Generalized anxiety disorder or other anxiety disorders
- Oppositional defiant disorder
- Panic disorder
- Personality disorders (narcissistic personality disorder, borderline personality disorder, antisocial personality disorder)
- Posttraumatic stress disorder
- Psychotic disorders (schizoaffective disorder, schizophrenia, and delusional disorder)
- Substance- or medication-induced mood disorder
- Substance-use disorder
- Unipolar MDD or persistent depressive disorder

SCREENING TOOLS

Because there are no laboratory tests specific to depression, clinicians can conduct depression screenings that use reliable and valid instruments to detect the presence or absence of symptoms, make a formal diagnosis, assess changes in symptom severity, and monitor client outcomes.

RISK ASSESSMENT PRACTICE CONSIDERATIONS

- Inquire about previous treatments, such as medication, and responses.
- Ask about family treatments and responses.
- Due to elevated risks in individuals with BD, thorough assessments of suicide risk, self-harm, substance use, and eating disorders should take place at each encounter.
- According to Yatham et al. (2018) and Goldstein et al. (2017), validated self-report instruments may be used as a screening to flag patients for bipolarity and can be part of an evidence-based approach to diagnose and inform next steps; however, more detailed assessments are required for diagnosis.
- If a baseline screening is initiated, repeat throughout the course of treatment to track and evaluate initial symptoms and response to treatment.

PEDIATRIC SCREENING TOOLS

- Affective Reactivity Index
- Child Behavior Checklist (pediatric BD phenotype)
- Child Depression Rating Scale Revised
- Child Mania Rating Scale and its 10-item short form
- General Behavior Inventory
- Kiddie Schedule for Affective Disorders and Schizophrenia for school-age children, Present and Lifetime version
- Mood Disorder Questionnaire
- The Achenbach Externalizing Scale
- The Child Behavior Checklist
- The Modified Overt Aggression Scale
- The Parent General Behavior Inventory
- The Rapid Mood Screener
- Young Mania Rating Scale

ADULT AND OLDER ADULT SCREENING TOOLS

- Altman Mania Rating Scale
- Beck Depression Inventory for Primary Care
- Bipolar Depression Rating Scale
- Bipolar Spectrum Diagnostic Scale

- Clinical Institute Withdrawal Assessment of Alcohol Scale, Revised
- Hypomania Checklist
- Hypomania Interview Guide
- Mood Disorder Questionnaire
- The Beck Scale for Suicidal Ideation
- The Patient Health Questionnaire – 9 Item (PHQ-9)
- The Rapid Mood Screener
- The "Two-Question Screen" (PHQ-2)

ORGANIC ETIOLOGIES FOR BIPOLAR DISORDER

- Human immunodeficiency virus
- Hyperthyroidism (mania; may induce mood cycling)
- Metabolic disorders (hypoglycemia, hyperglycemia, Cushing's disease, Addison's disease)
- Organic brain syndromes (multiple sclerosis, frontal lobe dementia, epilepsy)
- Thyroid disease (hypothyroidism [lethargy] or depression)
- Tumor or lesion(s)
- Vitamin deficiency (B_{12} deficiency)

OTHER LABORATORY MONITORING CONSIDERATIONS

- Bone mineral density
  - Baseline in older adults and follow-up as clinically indicated
- Blood pressure
  - Baseline, 1 month and with dose changes
- Electrocardiogram
  - Baseline and dose changes
  - Monitor children and older adults with more caution
  - Body mass index
  - Baseline, repeat 4 to 6 weeks and repeat in 6 months
- Electrolytes
  - Baseline, repeat 4 to 6 weeks and repeat in 6 months
  - Monitor older adults for hyponatremia with more caution
  - Assess fall risk due to hypotension
- Pregnancy test (if applicable)
- Suicidality
  - Baseline, daily, weekly, monthly, or variable depending on clinical presentation
- Thyroid tests
  - Baseline and follow-up as clinically indicated
- Vitamin D, B_{12}, folate
  - Baseline and if clinically indicated
- Screen for prevalence of potentially medication or substance use
  - Urine drug screen for stimulants and other substances

- Screen for prevalence of potentially inappropriate medication in older adults
  - Associated with increased morbidity, mortality, and decrease in quality of life
  - Screening Tool in Older Persons' Prescriptions
  - Beers Criteria
- Thyroid tests
  - Baseline and follow-up as clinically indicated

Essential Facts

When to consider mixed features using "the four A's":

- Anxiety
- Agitation
- Anger/irritability
- Attentional disturbance—distractibility

(McIntyre et al., 2020)

DIAGNOSTIC CHALLENGES

BD is an affective disorder that is characterized by cyclical and fluctuating changes in energy and disinhibition and is associated with characteristic cognitive, physical, and behavioral symptoms that impair the patient's interpersonal and/or occupational functioning; however, the presentation for BD can vary (Dome et al., 2019). Many individuals with BP-I experience one or more depressed or mixed episodes, even though these episodes are not required for diagnosis. Many individuals with BD typically seek help during depressive episodes (or mixed features) rather than periods of mania; therefore, it can be particularly challenging for clinicians to differentiate between unipolar and bipolar depression.

Clinical differentiation between BD and borderline personality disorder (BPD) can also be difficult due to an overlap of symptom domains. Both conditions may include impulsivity, mood lability, and affective instability; therefore, during the diagnostic interview, the use of validated self-report standardized screening instruments may be helpful to diagnose these disorders accurately (Palmer et al., 2021). Additionally, BP-II can also be challenging to diagnose because the symptoms of hypomania may not present or be reported to clinicians by patients, caregivers, or other collateral sources. Furthermore, hypomania can be mistaken as a "normal" state and not be seen as the cause of functionality (APA, 2013; Kelly, 2018).

The *DSM-5* notes that the typical onset of cyclothymic disorder is in adolescence or early adulthood, though it can appear in children. Cyclothymic disorder often goes underdiagnosed or misdiagnosed in children, adolescents, and adults because many of its features overlap with other conditions

(APA, 2013). Cyclothymic disorder usually has an insidious onset, and, due to the timing of onset, it can be difficult to tell whether mood symptoms are normal because youths are prone to hormonal fluctuations, labile mood, and overreacting to minor stressors and disappointments (APA, 2013). For example, mania in the adolescent is often atypical, with symptoms of irritability and flight of ideas appearing more frequently than euphoria and grandiosity; thus, cyclothymic disorder can easily be incorrectly diagnosed as another condition with similar features. In children, symptoms of ADHD and depression include irritability, restlessness, moodiness, and distractibility, which are also symptoms associated with cyclothymia. According to Van Meter and Youngstrom (2012), mood instability and irritability are symptoms in conditions such as cyclothymia, BPD, atypical depression, other specified bipolar and related disorders, unspecified bipolar and related disorders, substance abuse disorders, substance/medication-induced bipolar and related disorders, and bipolar and related disorders due to another medical condition. All of these conditions share similar diagnostic features, making it difficult for clinicians to decipher key diagnostic points. Medical conditions such as hypothyroidism or hyperthyroidism can produce mood cycling and should also be considered for these individuals.

CLINICAL PRESENTATION FOR CHILDREN AND ADOLESCENTS WITH BIPOLAR DISORDER

The diagnosis of BD in childhood and adolescence has been controversial within the field of mental health, with the exact clinical characteristics of pediatric BD in question among experts (Goldstein et al., 2017). Although irritability and mania are the most common symptoms in pediatric BD, to meet diagnostic criteria, the child must experience severe shifts in conjunction with the presence of episodic manic symptoms such as fluctuations in energy and/or sleep (Goldstein et al., 2017). According to Birmaher et al. (2009), in adolescent groups with bipolar spectrum disorders, depression was the most common initial symptom that was later followed by mania or hypomania. Moreover, children were more likely to have had subsyndromal manic/hypomanic symptoms as their first episode (Birmaher et al., 2009).

Chronic course of extreme shifts in mood, mania, hypomania, depression, irritability, unstable moodiness, or mixed symptoms of depression and mania with rapid cycles and temper outbursts are associated with pediatric and adolescent BD. Challenges with diagnosis are attributed to overlapping diagnostic features with ADHD, disruptive mood dysregulation disorder, and other oppositional behaviors. In addition, children and adolescents may have difficulties expressing their symptoms compared to adults; therefore, it is important that clinicians distinguish age-appropriate conduct and behaviors from behaviors that exceed what is expected in each developmental stage (Goldstein et al., 2017). Symptom sequence can help clinicians differentiate BD from some other disorders; therefore, a detailed history with a longitudinal course of symptoms along with parent, youth, and teacher reports on symptom checklists can guide diagnostic accuracy and decision-making for children with BD.

Essential Facts

In adolescents, the initial clinical presentation more closely resembles the presentation seen in adults.

CLINICAL PRESENTATION FOR ADULTS AND OLDER ADULTS WITH BIPOLAR DISORDER

Bipolar or related disorders should be considered for anyone who presents with depression, hypomania, mania, psychosis, and significant fluctuations in mood, energy, activity, behavior, sleep, and irritability. According to Kim et al. (2019), symptom severity may differ between individuals in terms of the duration and frequency of episodes, functional recovery after remission, and patterns of polarity.

Clinicians should collect patients' psychiatric history and conduct a mental status examination to assess patients for BD. It is important that clinicians gather data and evaluate patients' lifetime history and patterns of mood episodes and consider more than the current presenting problem to establish a diagnosis. Previous medical records, family observations, subjective history, and direct observation of symptoms are required for diagnostic accuracy. Additional challenges may include (a) lack of insight into illness (an individual's insight into their condition can be worse with BP-II than BP-I); (b) misunderstanding descriptions of terms used to describe mood symptoms, such as euphoria, up, elevated, expansive, overly happy, exuberant, and racing thoughts; (c) denial (patient or caregivers); and (d) stigma associated with mental illness.

According to the *DSM-5* (APA, 2013), onset of BD may occur through the fifth, sixth, and seventh decades of life. The initial onset of manic symptoms (e.g., sexual or social disinhibition) in mid-to-late life should prompt clinicians to consider medical conditions (neurologic or neuroendocrine problems) and require a medical work-up to assess for possible infectious etiologies, frontotemporal neurocognitive disorders, or substance use (steroid) withdrawal.

Use of alcohol and/or drugs such as stimulants is comorbid with manic, hypomanic, or pseudo-rebound depressive mood changes that can cloud the diagnostic picture. Stimulants, levodopa, and corticosteroids are the most commonly prescribed medications associated with secondary mania. These drugs may mimic manic symptoms and should decrease with drug clearance, therefore using about five half-lives as the relevant interval (and the longest half-life stated in a range). To ensure an accurate diagnosis, continue to monitor for possible substance with urine drug toxin screenings. Results of urine toxin screenings should remain negative for approximately 6 months before considering a mood disorder diagnosis. After assessing for safety (medical condition, drug use, etc.), antimanic medications (oral tablets, oral disintegrating tablets [ODTs], or intramuscular) with a fast onset of action are required for individuals experiencing acute mania (Goodwin et al., 2016).

Essential Facts

In older adults, syndromes of delirium and dementia often present difficulties in accurate diagnosis. An increased prevalence of depressive episodes is found in older adults versus younger adults with BD (Sajatovic et al., 2015).

U.S. FOOD AND DRUG ADMINISTRATION APPROVED FOR CHILDREN FOR BIPOLAR DISORDER MAINTENANCE

The United States Food and Drug Administration (FDA) approved second-generation antipsychotic (SGA) drugs for the treatment of acute mania and/or mixed mania in children and adolescents (10–17 years).

Risperidone (Risperdal, Risperdal Consta, Perseris)

U.S. Food and Drug Administration Approval

- Children and adolescents
- Thirteen years or older for schizophrenia
- Ten years or older for bipolar mania
- Five years or older for irritability associated with autism

Dosage Forms

- Tablets
- ODT (ODT can be used as an alternative for individuals who have difficulty swallowing tablets)
- Liquid
- IM, depot (Consta)**
- Perseris is a long-acting form (SQ; efficacy of IM and SQ dose not established in those younger than 18 years of age)
- Dosing for schizophrenia and bipolar mania
- Dosing for irritability associated with autism

Aripiprazole (Abilify)

U.S. Food and Drug Administration Indication

- Schizophrenia in those 13 years old or older
- Bipolar mania/acute mania in those 10 years old or older
- Tourette disorder in those 6 years old or older
- Autism associated with irritability in those 6 years old or older
    - Increase dose in 7-day increments until desired effect is reached.

Dosage Forms

- Tablet

**Treatment initiation recommendation for risperidone naïve patients, includes establishing tolerability with immediate release oral formulations of risperidone prior to initiating treatment with RISPERDAL CONSTA. If patient is stabilized on a fixed dose of oral risperidone for 2 weeks or more, then follow medication conversion recommendations based on dosage. Patients should be closely monitored during the treatment initiation period.

- ODT (ODT can be used as an alternative for individuals who have difficulty swallowing tablets)
- Oral solution

Olanzapine (Zyprexa, Symbyax, Zyprexa Relprevv [Olanzapine Pamoate])

U.S. Food and Drug Administration Approval

- Schizophrenia in those 13 years old and older
- Bipolar mania/acute mania in those13 years old and older

Dosage Forms

- Oral tablets
- ODT
- IM (safety of the IM form is not established in those younger than 18 years old)
- Depot
- Combination olanzapine-fluoxetine capsule (safety is not established in those younger than 18 years old in bipolar mania)

Olanzapine–Fluoxetine Combination (OFC) in Bipolar Depression (Symbyax)

U.S. Food and Drug Administration Approval

- FDA approved fluoxetine/olanzapine (Symbyax) in 2003 for the treatment of BD (Rhee et al., 2020).
- FDA indication is for BD depression in youth aged 10 to 17 years old.

Dosage Forms

- OFC capsule (mg equivalent olanzapine/mg equivalent fluoxetine)

Dosing in Bipolar Depression

- Increase dose based on efficacy and tolerability.

Second-Generation Antipsychotics (SGAs; Refer to Chapter 7 for More on SGA Management)

- Monitoring for specific medications (e.g., weight and lipid profile, growth)
- Extrapyramidal symptoms
- Hyperprolactinemia
- Metabolic side effects
- Monitor neutrophil count
  - Suspend medication if absolute neutrophil count falls below 1,000/mm^3

Paliperidone (Invega, Invega Sustenna, Invega Trinza, Xeplion, Trevicta)

U.S. Food and Drug Administration Approval

- Schizophrenia in those 12 years old and older

Dosage Forms

- Extended-release oral tablets
- One-month IM injection (efficacy of IM dose not established in those younger than 18 years of age)

- Prior to initiation of monthly IM therapy, tolerability should be established with oral paliperidone or oral risperidone.
- Three-month IM injection (efficacy of IM dose not established in those younger than 18 years of age)
  - Prior to initiation of monthly IM therapy, tolerability should be established with oral paliperidone or oral risperidone.

Special Considerations in the Prescribing of Paliperidone

- Use with caution for individuals with preexisting gastrointestinal-narrowing disorders or gastrointestinal-tract alterations because drug is contained in a nondeformable controlled-release formulation.
- Swallow capsule and avoid crushing or chewing medication to avoid rapid bioavailability of paliperidone.
- Following drug release/absorption, the shell is expelled in stool.
- Monitor neutrophil count:
  - Suspend medication if absolute neutrophil count falls below 1,000/mm^3.

Quetiapine, Quetiapine XR (Seroquel, Seroquel XR)

Dosage Forms

- Tablets
- Extended-release tablets
  - Avoid chewing or crushing; swallow whole because Quetiapine XR is controlled release.

U.S. Food and Drug Administration Approval

- Schizophrenia in those 13 years old or older

Immediate Release

- May be divided into three doses per day.
- Continue therapy at lowest dose needed to maintain remission.

Extended Release

- Continue therapy at lowest dose needed to maintain remission
- Bipolar disorder/acute mania in those 10 years old or older.
- Immediate-release tablets:
  - Daily doses may also be divided into 3 doses per day.
  - Continue therapy at lowest dose needed to maintain remission.
- Extended-release tablets:
  - Daily doses may also be divided into 3 doses per day.
  - Continue therapy at lowest dose needed to maintain remission.

How to Switch From Immediate Release to Extended Release

- Convert from immediate-release to extended-release tablets at the equivalent total daily dose and administer once daily.
- Assess for individual dosage adjustments that may be required.

Special Considerations for Quetiapine

- If quetiapine has been discontinued:
  - If more than 1 week discontinued, retitrate using the initial dosing schedule.
  - If less than 1 week discontinued, restart on their previous maintenance dose.
- Extended-release formulation: Do not break, chew, or crush.
  - Swallow whole since drug is sustained release.

PRESCRIBING CONSIDERATIONS FOR CHILDREN AND ADOLESCENTS FOR SECOND-GENERATION ANTIPSYCHOTICS

- Injectable formulations are not approved in children/adolescents.
- Monitor weight at baseline and every 3 months ongoing.
- Screen for personal and family history of diabetes; obesity and issues with blood pressure, fasting plasma glucose, fasting lipid profile, dyslipidemia, waist circumference, hypertension, and cardiovascular disease.
- Monitor absolute neutrophil count (stop if below 1,000/mm^3).
- Assess for tardive dyskinesia.
- If mild side effects, wait to see tolerance and determine risk versus benefit of continuing the medication.

Asenapine (Saphris)

Dosage Forms

- Sublingual (SL)
  - The medication must be prescribed SL in children.
  - For absorption to occur, patients cannot eat or drink × 10 minutes after administering medication.

U.S. Food and Drug Administration Approval

- Acute mania/mixed mania in those 10 years old and older
- SL:
  - Daily doses are divided into 2 doses per day.
  - Continue therapy at the lowest dose needed to maintain remission.
  - Use SGAs (refer to Chapter 7 for more on SGA management).
  - Monitor for specific medications (e.g., weight and lipid profile, growth).
  - Review extrapyramidal symptoms.
  - Consider hyperprolactinemia.
  - Watch for metabolic side effects.
  - Monitor neutrophil count.
  - Suspend medication if absolute neutrophil count falls below 1,000/mm^3.

Lurasidone (Latuda)

U.S. Food and Drug Administration Approval

- Bipolar depression (Latuda, ages 10 and older, monotherapy)
- Bipolar depression (Latuda, adjunct)
- Schizophrenia (Latuda, ages 13 and older)

Dosage Forms

- Tablet

Dosing Considerations

- Monitor weight, metabolic functions, blood pressure, fasting plasma glucose, and fasting lipid profile using the pediatric height/weight chart.
- Use with caution if there is a personal and family history of diabetes, obesity, dyslipidemia, hypertension, and cardiovascular disease.

Essential Facts

Mood stabilizer categories have been established, with euthymia being the baseline mood; therefore, Class A mood stabilizers are defined as stabilizing mood from *above* baseline (euthymia), and Class B mood stabilizers as stabilizing mood from *below* baseline (euthymia; Grunze et al., 2021).

MOOD STABILIZERS

Lithium is considered the most stabilizing and most effective drug for the treatment of recurrent depressive disorders and BDs. Lithium has a low risk of worsening depression and inducing mania. With proper surveillance, lithium is prescribed in pediatrics and during postpartum because of its neuroprotective properties, slow onset of action, and lower side-effect risk profile (Goodwin et al., 2016).

Lithium

U.S. Food and Drug Administration Approval

- FDA indication for the treatment and recurrence/prevention of mania in youths aged 12 years and older.
- Lithium-specific considerations: Lithium is well known for its antisuicide effects.
- Prior to starting lithium, baseline tests include:
  - Blood urea nitrogen
  - Creatinine electrolytes
  - Thyrotropin (thyroid-stimulating hormone)
  - Electrocardiogram
  - Urine pregnancy test should be obtained prior to initiating lithium. Continue to monitor lithium's potential effects on kidney, thyroid gland, and heart functioning. Assess for tremors, gastrointestinal side effects, and skin conditions such as acne.

Monitoring Lithium in Children and Older Adults

- Lithium has a very low therapeutic index; that is, a low ratio between the dose (or serum level) that is associated with toxicity (primarily CNS and renal toxicity) and the dose associated with therapeutic effect.

- Check serum concentrations after 5 consecutive days of taking medication.
- It is measured 4 to 7 days after initiating medication and after each dose change.
- Ideally, lithium levels are drawn approximately 12 hours after the last dose (12-hour serum trough level the morning before the first dose of the day).
- Monitor lithium plasma levels weekly × 2 weeks, then every 2 to 3 months; after a stable lithium dose is achieved, lithium serum concentrations are measured every 3 to 6 months regularly.
  - Doses are titrated up by 300 mg/day every 4 to 7 days (depending upon response, tolerability, serum levels).
  - The target serum concentration is 0.6 to 1.4 mEq/L (0.6–1.4 mmol/L).
  - Minimum effective lithium level for all age groups should be 0.40 mmol/L.
  - Doses of immediate-release preparations are given in two or three divided doses.
  - Extended-release preparations are usually given twice per day (or once daily).

Lithium and Older Adults

Older adults are more prone to acute lithium toxicity due to:

- Reduced renal clearance
  - For the older adult, a more conservative approach is suggested, usually 0.40 to 0.60 mEq/L, with the option to go to maximally 0.70 or 0.80 mEq/L at ages 65 to 79 years, and to maximally 0.70 mEq/L for those 80 years of age and above.
  - Individuals 50 years of age and older, with rapid cycling with the addition of lithium to valproate, are strongly suggestive for improvements in depression and prevention of suicide attempts and deaths.
- Vulnerability to medical comorbidity is present.
- Drug–drug interactions (for adults and older adults):
  - Angiotensin-converting enzyme inhibitors increase lithium level.
  - Calcium antagonists increase or decrease lithium level.
  - Thiazide and loop diuretics increase lithium level.
  - Nonsteroidal anti-inflammatory drugs increase lithium level.
  - Potassium-sparing diuretics decrease lithium level.

Treatment Resistance

- Lithium is recommended in children with (a) poor responses to multiple (2–3) trials of SGAs and (b) partial responses to SGAs as an adjunctive medication for 7 to 14 days while tapering down the SGA and titrating up the lithium dose (Goodwin et al., 2016).

Table 8.4 presents divalproex, lamotrigine, and valproate's indications and prescribing information.

Table 8.4

Mood Stabilizers

Generic Name (Brand Name)	Dosage Forms	FDA Approval	Clinical Considerations
Carbamazepine (Tegretol)	Extended-Release Capsules (Equetro, Carbatrol)	*Adults:* bipolar I disorder, epilepsy, trigeminal neuralgia *Non-FDA Uses:* dementia, alcohol withdrawal syndrome, behavioral syndrome *Off-Label:* restless leg syndrome, schizophrenia *Pediatrics:* epilepsy *Older Adult Considerations:* *,**	Generally used as a second-line agent and for individuals who are lithium nonresponders *Therapeutic blood level:* 4–12 μg per mL *Prescribing considerations:* Associated with drug–drug interactions related to induction of cytochrome P450 liver enzymes
Lamotrigine (Lamictal)	Tablets Chewable Tablets Oral Disintegrating Tablets Extended-Release Tablets	*Adults:* bipolar I disorder, epilepsy *Non-FDA Uses:* bipolar depression, unipolar depression, bipolar mania schizophrenia, neuropathic pain, MDD *Pediatrics:* adjunctive therapy, Lennox-Gastaut syndrome, partial seizure ages 2 and older, monotherapy for seizures age 16 and older *Off-Label:* bipolar I disorder (12 to 17 years) *Older Adult Considerations:* *	Enzyme-inducing antiepileptic (AED) drugs include carbamazepine, phenytoin phenobarbital, and primidone. Valproate inhibits lamotrigine metabolism. If medication is not taken for more than 5 days, start at initial titration dosing range. Instruct patients to not break, chew, or crush extended-release tablets. Psychoeducation: report any adverse symptoms associated with risk of life-threatening rash. Stevens-Johnson syndrome: discontinue medication and possible hospitalization.

*Start at the lowest dosage and titrate slowly while monitoring the patient for any side effects. Assess for mental status changes.

**May exacerbate or cause SIADH or hyponatremia; monitor sodium level closely when starting or changing dosages in older adults (Beers Criteria, 2019, p. 13).

(*continued*)

Table 8.4

Mood Stabilizers (*continued*)

Generic Name (Brand Name)	Dosage Forms	FDA Approval	Clinical Considerations
Lithium	IM Tablets IR Capsules Solution Extended-Release Tablets	*Adults:* bipolar I disorder, acute mania *Non-FDA Uses:* bipolar depression, depression, anti-suicide agent *Pediatrics:* acute mania; bipolar disorder (ages 7 and older) *Off-Label:* bipolar disorder (maintain serum lithium levels at 0.8–1.2 mEq/L) *Older Adult Considerations:* Lower plasma lithium doses are preferred (plasma levels 0.6 mEq/L) monitor for mental status changes assess for polydrug interactions*	Regular lithium levels are essential. A one-time evening dose may be considered once patient is stable. Use lowest lithium dose with adequate therapeutic response obtained. Lithium has a very low therapeutic index. Maintain serum lithium levels at 0.8–1.2 mEq/L). Minimum effective lithium level for all age groups should be 0.40 mmol/L. Lithium blood levels are measured 12 hours after the last evening dose ("trough" level). Monitor lithium plasma levels weekly × 2 weeks, then every 3 months, once stable, every 6 to 12 months.
Oxcarbazepine (Trileptal, Oxtellar)	Film-Coated Tablets Extended-Release Tablets Oral Suspension	*Adults:* partial seizures, major adjunctive therapy in depressive disorder *Off-Label:* diabetic neuropathy, neuralgia/neuropathy, bipolar disorder *Non-FDA Uses:* anxiety *Pediatrics:* safety in pediatric use has not been established *Older Adult Considerations:* *,**	Associated with drug–drug interactions related to induction of cytochrome P450 liver enzymes. Monitor sodium levels due to risk of hyponatremia.

*Start at the lowest dosage and titrate slowly while monitoring the patient for any side effects. Assess for mental status changes.

**May exacerbate or cause SIADH or hyponatremia; monitor sodium level closely when starting or changing dosages in older adults (Beers Criteria, 2019, p. 13).

(*continued*)

Table 8.4

Mood Stabilizers (*continued*)

Generic Name (Brand Name)	Dosage Forms	FDA Approval	Clinical Considerations
Valproate (Depakote, Depakene, Stavzor, Depacon)	Capsules (Depakene) Delayed-Release Capsules/Tablets (Stavzor) Delayed-Release Sprinkle Capsules Depakene Syrup Extended-Release Tablets Injectable Solution (Depacon as Valproate Sodium)	*Adults:* bipolar mania, migraine prophylaxis, seizures *Non-FDA Uses:* bipolar depression, schizophrenia—adjunctive, diabetic neuropathy, peripheral neuralgia, status epilepticus, pathologic impulsivity/ aggression *Older Adult Considerations:* Lower plasma lithium doses are preferred*	May cause false positive in urine ketone test results. May alter results for thyroid function tests. May need to taper slowly off treatment to avoid symptoms of withdrawal. Divalproex IR may reduce GI side effects. Trough plasma drug levels in therapeutic range for valproate: 50–120 μg/mL. Levels are measured 12 hours after the last evening dose ("trough" level). Dosages to achieve therapeutic plasma levels can vary.
Topiramate (Topamax)	Tablet Extended-Release Capsule Sprinkle Capsule	*Adults:* seizures, seizures associated with Lennox-Gaustat syndrome, migraine headache prophylaxis, weight management *Off-Label:* bipolar disorder, neuroleptic weight gain, binge eating disorder, alcoholism *Pediatrics:* seizures, seizures associated with Lennox-Gaustat syndrome (2 years and older), migraine headache (12 years and older) *Older Adult Considerations:* *	Sprinkle capsule can be sprinkled over food (applesauce).

*Start at the lowest dosage and titrate slowly while monitoring the patient for any side effects. Assess for mental status changes.

FDA, U.S. Food and Drug Administration; GAD, general anxiety disorder; GI, gastrointestinal; MDD, major depressive disorder; OCD, obsessive-compulsive disorder; ODT, orally disintegrating tablet; PTSD, posttraumatic stress disorder

MEDICATIONS FOR ADULTS WITH BIPOLAR AND RELATED DISORDERS

No single agent is identified as the ideal mood stabilizer; therefore, additional anticonvulsant drugs used for mood stability are presented in Table 8.4, and neuropoietic drugs are presented in Chapter 7.

Mood Stabilizers

- Lithium
- Carbamazepine
- Oxcarbazepine
- Valproate
- Lamotrigine

Neuroleptics

- Cariprazine
- Aripiprazole
- Asenapine
- Olanzapine–monotherapy
- Quetiapine–monotherapy
- Ziprasidone
- Risperidone
- Lurasidone
- Brexpiprazole
- Haloperidol

MAINTENANCE PHASE OF TREATMENT

Treatment goals for BD and related disorders consist of bringing patients with mania or depression to symptomatic recovery and stable mood and reducing and preventing relapse, reducing hospital readmissions, and improving medication adherence. Combined psychosocial and pharmacologic treatments to manage BD relapse, suicidal behavior, and comorbid medical and substance use problems that contribute to cognitive, psychosocial, residential, and occupational impairments remain an ongoing clinical challenge.

Counseling and family psychotherapy are important components of management and should be encouraged to help individuals and families learn to identify and cope more effectively with warning signs of mood fluctuations. Psychotherapy options include (a) behavioral therapy to decrease stress, (b) cognitive behavioral therapy to learn to identify problem thinking and learn ways to modify thought processes, (c) group psychoeducation to make meaningful connections and support others, and (d) family-focused therapy to help with the development of coping skills to assist with stressors, social and school/occupational functioning, medication adherence, and development of support systems and other social supports.

Clients and family members should be educated on how to recognize warning signs of relapse, such as isolation or reckless behavior. Stress management, medication and treatment compliance, and limiting alcohol and caffeine intake can help prevent relapse. Clinicians should provide informational pamphlets and videos, offer community support, provide suicidal crisis telephone services, and offer intensive outpatient programs and patient advocacy groups to support individuals with BD.

ONGOING MONITORING

- Suicidality
- Signs of psychosis
- Mood swings
- Violence and self-harmful behaviors
- Sleep patterns
- Medication compliance
- Surveillance for possible comorbidities
- Alcohol and substance use
- Lab tests when indicated
- Sleep changes and sleep hygiene
- Diet and exercising patterns
- Caffeine intake
- Social and occupational functioning decline
- Assess for reckless behaviors that accompany mania (sexual, gambling, shopping, etc.)

CRITERIA FOR REFERRAL

- Always consider hospital admission if mania is diagnosed, especially if there are risks to the patient and/or others. Also consider potential dangers and risks associated with poor judgment and potential harm in areas of work, personal relationships, alcohol/drug use, spending, driving, and sexual activity (Goodwin et al., 2016).
- Consider referral if the patient has suicidal thoughts and/or has a recent history of suicide attempt(s).
- Consider referral if the patient has poor response to two adequate trials of medication and is beginning a third medication trial (Goodwin et al., 2016).
- Consider referral if the patient has a complicated psychiatric medication regimen or comorbid conditions (i.e., psychosis, drug dependency).
- Consider referral with adolescents due to potential risk factors.

SUMMARY

Patients often require lifelong treatment to alleviate negative outcomes of BD and to prevent relapse; therefore, it is important to set realistic monitoring benchmarks and recommendations. As mental health clinicians offer their expertise based on recent evidence, it is important to incorporate individual preferences into care. Patient-centered therapeutic approaches for individuals that include learning strategies of coping, improving interpersonal relationships, and management adherence should play a central role in treatment and management decisions through shared decision-making.

RESOURCES

- The National Institute of Mental Health: www.nimh.nih.gov/health/publications/bipolar-disorder-in-children-and-teens
- The American Academy of Child and Adolescent Psychiatry (AACAP): www.aacap.org
- The American Psychiatric Association: www.psychiatry.org
- Depression and Bipolar Support Alliance (DBSA): www.dbsalliance.org
- Help Guide: https://www.helpguide.org/articles/bipolar-disorder/helping-someone-with-bipolar-disorder.htm
- The National Alliance on Mental Illness or NAMI: www.nami.org/Home
- The International Society for Bipolar Disorders (ISBD): www.isbd.org

REVIEW QUESTIONS

1. Which one of the following statements about lithium is incorrect?
   a. Lithium is well known for its antisuicide effects.
   b. Lithium levels are drawn approximately 12 hours after the last dose (12-hour serum trough level).
   c. A baseline blood urea nitrogen, creatinine, electrolytes, thyroid function, and electrocardiogram and CT scan of the brain are required before starting lithium.
   d. The target lithium serum concentration is 0.6 to 1.4 mEq/L (0.6 to 1.4 mmol/L).
2. Children diagnosed with bipolar disorder (BD) are more likely to ______________________.
   a. Have a first-degree relative with BD
   b. Have a clearer clinical picture than adults with BD
   c. Take antidepressants and achieve optimal outcomes
   d. Have better treatment outcomes than adult-onset BD
3. Which one of the following is the most accurate regarding the use of screening tools in bipolar disorder (BD)?
   a. Reliable and valid instruments can be used to detect the presence or absence of symptoms, make a formal diagnosis, assess changes in symptom severity, and monitor client outcomes.
   b. Tools can be used to make a diagnosis of BD without the structural interview.
   c. Tools cannot be used for children because they would cloud the clinical picture.
   d. Tools can be used for mania but not for depression.
4. Which one of the following lists the four A's in mixed bipolar symptoms?
   a. Anxiety, agitation, anger/irritability, attentional disturbance–distractibility
   b. Anxiety, affective flattening, anger, anhedonia
   c. Anxiety, agitation, anhedonia, adherence to therapy
   d. Adherence to treatment, attention deficit and hyperactivity, anger, anhedonia

5. Cyclothymia can best be described as which one of the following?
   a. A simple condition for clinicians to diagnose because many of its features overlap with other conditions
   b. A condition that is difficult to diagnose as it may be mistaken for normal mood swings.
   c. A condition unable to be diagnosed in individuals under 18 years of age
   d. A diagnosis requiring at least one manic episode

REFERENCES

American Geriatrics Society Beers Criteria® Update Expert Panel (2019). American Geriatrics Society 2019 Updated AGS Beers Criteria® for Potentially Inappropriate Medication Use in Older Adults. *Journal of the American Geriatrics Society, 67*(4), 674–694. https://doi.org/10.1111/jgs.15767

American Psychiatric Association. (2013). *Diagnostic and statistical manual of mental disorders* (5th ed.). https://doi.org/10.1176/appi.books.9780890425596

Birmaher, B., Axelson, D., Strober, M., Gill, M. K., Yang, M., Ryan, N., Goldstein, B., Hunt, J., Esposito-Smythers, C., Iyengar, S., Goldstein, T., Chiapetta, L., Keller, M., & Leonard, H. (2009). Comparison of manic and depressive symptoms between children and adolescents with bipolar spectrum disorders. *Bipolar Disorders, 11*(1), 52–62. https://doi.org/10.1111/j.1399-5618.2008.00659.x

Dome, P., Rihmer, Z., & Gonda, X. (2019). Suicide risk in bipolar disorder: A brief review. *Medicina, 55*(8), Article 403. https://doi.org/10.3390/medicina55080403

Ferrari, A. J., Stockings, E., Khoo, J. P., Erskine, H. E., Degenhardt, L., Vos, T., & Whiteford, H. A. (2016). The prevalence and burden of bipolar disorder: Findings from the Global Burden of Disease Study 2013. *Bipolar Disorders, 18*(5), 440–450. https://doi.org/10.1111/bdi.12423

Goldstein, B. I., Birmaher, B., Carlson, G. A., DelBello, M. P., Findling, R. L., Fristad, M., Kowatch, R. A., Miklowitz, D. J., Nery, F. G., Perez-Algorta, G., Van Meter, A., Zeni, C. P., Correll, C. U., Kim, H. W., Wozniak, J., Chang, K. D., Hillegers, M., & Youngstrom, E. A. (2017). The International Society for Bipolar Disorders Task Force report on pediatric bipolar disorder: Knowledge to date and directions for future research. *Bipolar Disorders, 19*(7), 524–543. https://doi.org/10.1111/bdi.12556

Goodwin, G. M., Haddad, P. M., Ferrier, I. N., Aronson, J. K., Barnes, T. R. H., Cipriani, A., Coghill, D. R., Fazel, S., Geddes, J. R., Grunze, H., Holmes, E. A., Howes, O., Hudson, S., Hunt, N., Jones, I., Macmillan, I. C., McAllister-Williams, H., Miklowitz, D. R., … Young, A. H. (2016). Evidence-based guidelines for treating bipolar disorder: Revised third edition recommendations from the British Association for Psychopharmacology. *Journal of Psychopharmacology, 30*(6), 495–553. https://doi.org/10.1177/0269881116636545

Grunze, A., Amann, B. L., & Grunze, H. (2021). Efficacy of carbamazepine and its derivatives in the treatment of bipolar disorder. *Medicina, 57*(5), Article 433. https://doi.org/10.3390/medicina57050433

Hui Poon, S., Sim, K., & Baldessarini, R. J. (2015). Pharmacological approaches for treatment-resistant bipolar disorder. *Current Neuropharmacology, 13*(5), 592–604. https://doi.org/10.2174/1570159x13666150630171954

Kelly, T. (2018). Prospective: Is bipolar disorder being over diagnosed? *International Journal of Methods in Psychiatric Research, 27*(3), Article e1725. https://doi.org/10.1002/mpr.1725

Kim, K., Yang, H., Na, E., Lee, H., Jang, O. J., Yoon, H. J., Oh, H. S., Ham, B. J., Park, S. C., Lin, S. K., Tan, C. H., Shinfuku, N., & Park, Y. C. (2019). Examining patterns of polypharmacy in bipolar disorder: Findings from the REAP-BD, Korea. *Psychiatry Investigation*, *16*(5), 397–402. https://doi.org/10.30773/pi.2019.02.26.4

Maletic, V., & Raison, C. (2014). Integrated neurobiology of bipolar disorder. *Frontiers in Psychiatry*, *5*, Article 98. https://doi.org/10.3389/fpsyt.2014.00098

McIntyre, R. S., Berk, M., Brietzke, E., Goldstein, B. I., López-Jaramillo, C., Kessing, L. V., Malhi, G. S., Nierenberg, A. A., Rosenblat, J. D., Majeed, A., Vieta, E., Vinberg, M., Young, A. H., & Mansur, R. B. (2020). Bipolar disorders. *The Lancet*, *396*(10265), 1841–1856. https://doi.org/10.1016/S0140-6736(20)31544-0

Palmer, B. A., Pahwa, M., Geske, J. R., Kung, S., Nassan, M., Schak, K. M., Alarcon, R. D., Frye, M. A., & Singh, B. (2021). Self-report screening instruments differentiate bipolar disorder and borderline personality disorder. *Brain and Behavior*, *11*(7), Article e02201. https://doi.org/10.1002/brb3.2201

Rhee, T. G., Olfson, M., Nierenberg, A. A., & Wilkinson, S. T. (2020). 20-year trends in the pharmacologic treatment of bipolar disorder by psychiatrists in outpatient care settings. *The American Journal of Psychiatry*, *177*(8), 706–715. https://doi.org/10.1176/appi.ajp.2020.19091000

Sajatovic, M., Strejilevich, S. A., Gildengers, A. G., Dols, A., Al Jurdi, R. K., Forester, B. P., Kessing, L. V., Beyer, J., Manes, F., Rej, S., Rosa, A. R., Schouws, S. N., Tsai, S. Y., Young, R. C., & Shulman, K. I. (2015). A report on older-age bipolar disorder from the International Society for Bipolar Disorders Task Force. *Bipolar Disorders*, *17*(7), 689–704. https://doi.org/10.1111/bdi.12331

Van Meter, A. R., & Youngstrom, E. A. (2012). Cyclothymic disorder in youth: Why is it overlooked, what do we know and where is the field headed? *Neuropsychiatry*, *2*(6), 509–519. https://www.ncbi.nlm.nih.gov/pmc/articles/PMC3609426

Yatham, L. N., Kennedy, S. H., Parikh, S. V., Schaffer, A., Bond, D. J., Frey, B. N., Sharma, V., Goldstein, B. I., Rej, S., Beaulieu, S., Alda, M., MacQueen, G., Milev, R. V., Ravindran, A., O'Donovan, C., McIntosh, D., Lam, R. W., Vazquez, G., Kapczinski, F., … Berk, M. (2018). Canadian Network for Mood and Anxiety Treatments (CANMAT) and International Society for Bipolar Disorders (ISBD) 2018 guidelines for the management of patients with bipolar disorder. *Bipolar Disorders*, *20*(2), 97–170. https://doi.org/10.1111/bdi.12609

9

Stimulants/Neurodevelopmental Disorders

Neurodevelopmental disorders (NDs) are a group of acquired developmental conditions that impact both cognitive and social communicative development, including an individual's cognition, language, behavior, gross motor skills, interpersonal relationships, and organization skills. In turn, the impairment of these skills impacts personal, social, academic, and/or occupational functioning (Rosenblum et al., 2019). NDs are considered the most prevalent chronic medical condition encountered in pediatric primary care, and are typically diagnosed during infancy, childhood, or adolescence, with a chronic course of impairment generally lasting into adulthood.

In this chapter you will learn:

1. How to evaluate background information about attention deficit hyperactivity disorder (ADHD) and other neurodevelopmental disorders (NDs)
2. How to determine the common treatments for ADHD
3. How to compare pharmacologic options for ADHD and related disorders
4. How to name five key features of ADHD and related disorders
5. How to determine the appropriate screening tools for ADHD
6. How to consider medication and safety in prescribing for and managing ADHD and related disorders
7. How to assess therapeutic responses in ADHD and related disorders

According to the *Diagnostic and Statistical Manual of Mental Disorders* (5th ed.; *DSM-5*; American Psychiatric Association [APA], 2013), NDs can fall into the following categories: (a) intellectual disability (ID); (b) communication disorders (language disorder, speech sound disorder, childhood onset fluency disorder (stuttering), and social/pragmatic communication disorder); (c) autism spectrum disorder (ASD); (d) attention deficit hyperactivity disorder (ADHD; predominantly inattentive or hyperactive/impulsive); (e) specific learning disorder (involving reading, written expression, and/or mathematics); (f) motor disorders (developmental coordination disorder, stereotypic movement disorder, and tic disorders), and (g) other NDs (Savatt & Myers, 2021, p. 2). It is not uncommon for cognitive and language delays and ADHD to co-occur. For example, individuals with ASD frequently have an ID, and children with ADHD may have learning and language problems (APA, 2013; Wolraich et al., 2019).

ADHD is characterized by persistent and trans-situational patterns of age-inappropriate levels of inattention, hyperactivity, and impulsivity that interfere with normal development, personal functioning, and well-being (Franke et al., 2018). ADHD, the most common neurobehavioral disorder of childhood, affects children's academic achievement, social interactions, and overall well-being (Rosenblum et al., 2019; Wolraich et al., 2019). ADHD affects an estimated 5% to 12% of school-aged children and between 2.5% and 4.9% of adults (APA, 2013; Cortese et al., 2018; Klein et al., 2017; Robberecht et al., 2020). Although ADHD does not emerge in late adulthood and is often underdiagnosed in early adulthood, an estimated 3% of older adults have ADHD (Children and Adults with Attention-Deficit/Hyperactivity Disorder [CHADD], n.d.). Estimated annual incremental costs for ADHD in the United States range between \$143 billion and \$266 billion (Cortese et al., 2018).

Although the pathogenesis for ADHD is not fully understood and there are no biologic tests, the diagnosis for ADHD meets standard criteria for validity of a mental disorder (Faraone et al., 2021). Researchers hypothesize that frontal–subcortical dysfunction and a network of interrelated brain areas all contribute to deficits in executive functions, inattention, hyperactivity, restlessness, emotional dysregulation, and impulsivity (Bahn et al., 2020; Cortese et al., 2018). Although not diagnostic (APA, 2013), children with ADHD exhibit increased slow-wave electroencephalograms, reduced total brain volume on MRI, and possibly a delay in posterior to anterior cortical maturation. The neurotransmitters norepinephrine (NE) and dopamine (DA) are key players in controlling prefrontal brain functions to modulate cognitive control functions such as memory, planning, impulse inhibition, attention, executive function, problem-solving, and communication (Bahn et al., 2020; Xing et al., 2016).

Essential Facts

Self-regulation is the process of managing and directing one's actions, thoughts, and feelings toward a goal.

Interoception is the perception of sensations from inside the body or the ability to sense the internal state of the body. Interoception is considered the first step in being able to attach to self and self-regulate.

Essential Facts

In a study of over 5,700 children, Faraone et al. (2021) found no significant differences among children with high, average, or low IQ and ADHD for individuals that met ADHD criteria.

Essential Facts

Common Comorbid Attention Deficit Hyperactivity Disorders

Common comorbid ADHD disorders include:

- Anxiety disorder
- ASD
- Bipolar disorder
- Conduct disorder
- Depression
- Developmental coordination disorder
- Learning disability
- Oppositional defiant disorder
- Personality disorders
- Sleep disorders
- Substance use disorders

Essential Facts

Approximately 80% of adults with attention deficit hyperactivity have one or more coexisting psychiatric disorders (Katzman et al., 2017).

Essential Facts

The first known description of attention deficit was published in 1775 by German physician Melchior Adam Weikard, who described how sensory stimuli captured the patient's attention and diverted the patient from their thoughts (Morris-Rosendahl & Crocq, 2020).

According to Bahn et al. (2020), functional impairments can vary throughout different stages of development because older children learn how to better control their impulses and self-regulate their behaviors. Self-regulation, a neuropsychological skill that develops from infancy through late adolescence, enables individuals to monitor and control thoughts, emotions, and behaviors (Tetering et al., 2020). Hyperactive and impulsive symptoms associated with ADHD tend to decline in adolescence, whereas inattentive symptoms tend to persist throughout adulthood (Bahn et al., 2020; Holbrook et al., 2016). Functional impairments induced by inattentive symptoms are more likely to be prominent later in life, such as in adolescence or adulthood, than in childhood, where motor hyperactivity is more apparent. In adults, ADHD can lead to substantial impairments, including traffic accidents, increased healthcare expenses, alcohol and substance use disorders, unemployment, interpersonal difficulties, risky behaviors, and premature death (Faraone et al., 2019; Franke et al., 2018; Tetering et al., 2020). This chapter provides an overview of ADHD and related NDs, and explores the key features, evidence in assessing, and how to diagnose, treat, and manage these conditions across the life span.

DIAGNOSTIC CRITERIA FOR ATTENTION DEFICIT HYPERACTIVITY DISORDER

A comprehensive and systematic clinical evaluation is required for individuals who present with inattention, hyperactivity, and/or impulsivity. Comprehensive evaluations address multiple factors, such as the patient's lifetime history of symptoms and impairments (in adults, symptoms prior to 12 years of age to symptoms at the current age); observer reports in several contexts; interviews with parents (and child, if possible; a detailed developmental, medical, and psychiatric history); ADHD screening assessment tools; past and current record reviews; and additional information from collateral informants on family functioning, peer relationships, and academic history. According to Wolraich et al. (2019), children or adolescents (ages 4 through 17) who present to a primary care clinical area with academic or behavioral difficulties in addition to symptoms of inattention, hyperactivity, or impulsivity require screening for ADHD. Critical components for diagnosis include chronicity, pervasiveness, and the degree of impairment. For example, symptoms must be present in individuals at 12 years of age and younger for at least 6 months in at least two different settings and must not be better explained by another disorder. Additionally, six out of nine possible inattentive symptoms (such as inability to pay attention to details or being distracted easily), and/or six out of nine possible hyperactivity/impulsivity symptoms (such as being "on the go" or difficulty waiting their turn) must be met to be diagnosed with ADHD. In adolescents and adults, the number of symptoms per category is reduced to five out of nine (APA, 2013; Storebø et al., 2018). The following is a summary of the diagnostic criteria for ADHD:

- Symptoms were present before the age of 12.
- Six symptoms in children ages 16 and younger and five symptoms in adolescents and adults ages 17 and older of inattention and/or of hyperactivity/impulsivity that have persisted for 6 months or longer to a degree that is inconsistent with developmental level and negatively impacts social and academic/occupational activities.
- Consistent pattern of inattentiveness or hyperactivity/impulsiveness were present before the age of 12 years old.

- Consistent pattern of inattentive or hyperactive/impulsive behaviors is present in two or more settings that interfere with home, school, or work activities.
- Symptoms negatively impact and/or reduce the quality of social, academic, or occupational functioning.
- Symptoms are not a result of another mental disorder, intoxication, or withdrawal of a substance.

These diagnostic criteria describe three different subtypes based on the following predominant symptoms: (a) predominantly inattentive type, (b) predominantly hyperactive–impulsive type, and (c) combined type: a combination of both hyperactive–impulsive and inattentive symptoms. An individual who does not clearly fit into one of those categories can be referred to as ADHD-Not Otherwise Specified. Additionally, continual assessment is required because symptoms and presentation can change over time. Table 9.1 lists the behavioral features commonly associated with ADHD, and Table 9.2 lists the key features of NDs.

Essential Facts

Predominantly inattentive presentation:

- Enough symptoms are present that meet the inattention diagnostic criteria, but not the hyperactivity–impulsivity category over the past 6 months.

Predominantly hyperactivity–impulsive presentation:

- Enough symptoms are present that meet the hyperactivity–impulsivity diagnostic criteria, but not inattention category over the past 6 months.

Essential Facts

The median age of ADHD diagnosis is 7 years of age.

DIAGNOSING ATTENTION DEFICIT HYPERACTIVITY DISORDER IN OLDER ADULTS

Older adults with ADHD have a long and consistent pattern of difficulties all related to maintaining focus and concentration. Clinicians should inquire about sleep and caffeine intake and obtain information from collateral sources. Because no specific screening tool has been developed for older adults, the six-question ADHD-ASRS Screener v1.1 and 18-question ADHD–ASRS Symptoms Checklist v1.1 can be used as part of the evaluation.

Diagnosing ADHD in older adults can be challenging due to lack of formal training for professionals and presenting symptoms that are similar to

Table 9.1

Features of Inattentive, Hyperactivity, and Impulsivity in ADHD

Subtype	Features
Predominantly inattentive: ▪ Six or more symptoms of inattention for children up to age 16 ▪ Five or more for adolescents aged 17 years and older and adults ▪ Symptoms of inattention that are inappropriate for developmental level have been present for at least 6 months	▪ Often fails to give close attention to details or makes careless mistakes in schoolwork, at work, or with other activities ▪ Often has difficulties holding attention on tasks or play activities ▪ Often does not seem to listen when spoken to directly ▪ Often does not follow through on instructions and fails to finish schoolwork, chores, or duties in the workplace (e.g., loses focus, side-tracked) ▪ Struggles with organizing tasks and activities ▪ Often avoids, dislikes, or is reluctant to do tasks that require mental effort over a long period of time (such as schoolwork or homework) ▪ Often loses things necessary for tasks and activities (e.g., school materials, pencils, books, tools, wallets, keys, paperwork, eyeglasses, mobile telephones) ▪ Distracted easily ▪ Forgetful
Predominantly hyperactivity and impulsivity: ▪ Six or more symptoms of hyperactivity–impulsivity for children up to age 16 years	▪ Restlessness, fidgets with or taps hands or feet, or squirms in seat ▪ Continuous activity; leaves seat in situations when remaining seated is expected
▪ Five or more for adolescents aged 17 years and older and adults ▪ Symptoms of hyperactivity–impulsivity that are disruptive and inappropriate for the individual's developmental level have been present for at least 6 months	▪ Often runs about or climbs in situations where it is not appropriate (adolescents or adults may be limited to feeling restless) ▪ Tends to always be active or unable to play or take part in leisure activities quietly ▪ Frequently "on the go"; acting as if "driven by a motor" ▪ Overly talkative, verboseness ▪ Impatiently blurts out an answer before a question has been completed ▪ Intolerantly struggles with waiting their turn ▪ Interjects or intrudes on others (e.g., intrudes into conversations or games)
Combined presentation	Enough symptoms of both criteria, inattention, and hyperactivity–impulsivity, were present for the past 6 months

ADHD, attention deficit hyperactivity disorders.

Table 9.2

Key Features of Neurodevelopmental Disorders

Disorder	Key Features
ASD ▪ Specify with or without intellectual impairment and with or without language impairment ▪ Associated with a known medical/genetic condition or environmental factor	▪ Deficits in social–emotional communication, verbal and nonverbal communication, and behaviors ▪ Inability to maintain and understand social contexts across multiple settings
ID (intellectual developmental disorder): ▪ Global developmental delay ▪ Unspecified ID (ID disorder)	▪ Limitations in intelligence and adaptive skills that impact at least one of three adaptive domains: conceptual, social, and practical ▪ Children <5 years old who fail to meet expected developmental milestones in several areas of intellectual functioning ▪ Deficits in problem-solving, reasoning, planning, abstract thinking, judgment, learning, development for personal independence ▪ Requiring ongoing support due to adaptive deficits
Communication disorders: ▪ Language disorder ▪ Speech sound disorder ▪ Child-onset fluency disorder (stuttering) ▪ Social (pragmatic) communication disorder ▪ Unspecified communication disorder	▪ Difficulties in the attainment, use, and expression of language (spoken, written, nonverbal communication, fluency, patterning of speech, etc.)
Specific learning disorder	▪ Educational skills are significantly lower than expected according to age, thus considerably affecting success and daily activities related to school or professional life (e.g., reading, writing, math, listening, speaking, reasoning)
Motor disorders: ▪ Developmental coordination disorder ▪ Stereotypic movement disorder ▪ Tic disorders ▪ Other specified tic disorder ▪ Unspecified tic disorder	▪ Deficits in obtaining, executing, and coordinating motor skills; overall developmental coordination is below or delayed for their chronological age
▪ Other ND: Unspecified NDs	▪ Symptoms are characteristic of an ND; however, symptoms do not meet the full criteria for any of the disorders in the ND diagnostic class but cause impairment in social, occupational, or other important areas of functioning

ASD, autism spectrum disorder; ND, neurodevelopmental disorder.

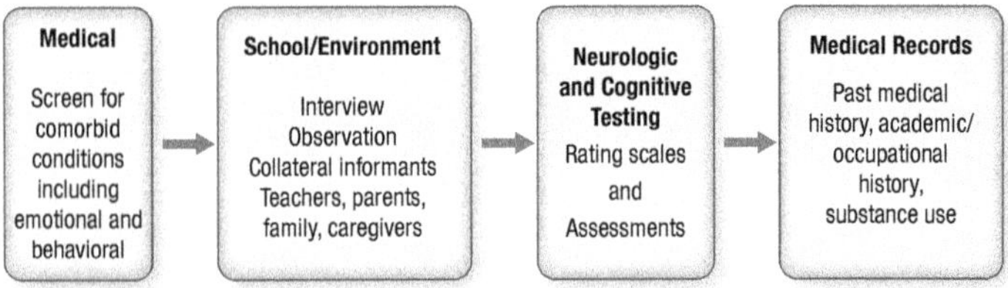

Figure 9.1 The components of a comprehensive evaluation.

dementia or mild cognitive impairments. It is important to inquire about poor sleep patterns, nutritional habits, caffeine intake, and any long-standing history of inattentiveness.

Medical professionals must conduct a comprehensive evaluation when assessing older adults for ADHD. Figure 9.1 represents the various components of a comprehensive evaluation.

Essential Facts

The prefrontal cortex (PFC) is the area of the brain most affected in patients with ADHD. The PFC is the area of the brain that regulates attention by sustaining focus while reducing distractibility (Sallee, 2010).

Untreated ADHD can cause problems throughout life. Some of the complications associated with untreated ADHD may include:

- Drug and alcohol use
- Financial problems
- Legal problems
- Poor occupation performance
- Poor school performance
- Problems with interpersonal relationships

Symptoms of ADHD can be subtle and resemble other illnesses; therefore, it is important to consider other conditions that could be behind a person's symptoms, such as the following:

- Anxiety disorders
- ASD
- Bipolar disorder
- Brain injury
- Child neglect or abuse
- Depressive disorders
- Disruptive mood dysregulation disorder
- Dysthymic disorder
- Hearing or visual impairment
- ID (intellectual developmental disorder)
- Intermittent explosive disorder

- Lead toxicity
- Malnutrition
- Mania
- Medication-induced side effects
- Medication-induced symptoms of ADHD
- Neurocognitive disorders
- Oppositional defiant disorder
- Other NDs
- Personality disorders
- Psychotic disorders
- Reactive attachment disorder
- Specific learning disorder
- Substance intoxication
- Substance use disorders

ATTENTION DEFICIT HYPERACTIVITY DISORDER DIAGNOSTIC CHALLENGES

During a clinical assessment, ADHD is considered when high levels of symptoms hinder an individual's social, academic, or occupational functioning, and a detailed developmental childhood history is needed that can sometimes be difficult to maintain (Bahn et al., 2020). Additionally, ADHD symptoms tend to change through developmental stages, which can complicate the clinical picture. For example, younger children display externalizing symptoms by exhibiting hyperactive–impulsive behaviors. In middle childhood and adolescence, inattentiveness, learning problems, failure to complete work, forgetfulness, depression, anxiety, and disorganization may also present without externalizing behaviors and persist through adulthood (Franke et al., 2018; Solanto, 2000). Although late-onset ADHD without any childhood history has been reported, future research is needed because it can be difficult to distinguish late-onset ADHD from other mental disorders (Bahn et al., 2020). Additional ADHD diagnostic challenges include the following:

- High rates of comorbidity can confuse presentation symptoms, which may overlap with other psychiatric disorders.
- Children under age 6 may present with ADHD symptoms; however, it may be difficult to observe their symptoms across multiple settings (as required by the *DSM-5*) if they do not attend a preschool or childcare program.
- ADHD, predominantly inattentive type, may not include hyperactivity among its features and go untested.
- It may be difficult to obtain teacher reports for adolescents, because many adolescents have multiple teachers.
- Interpatient response to each medication class can vary as the response to one class does not predict response to another.
- Individuals with ADHD are not always the best historians.
    - In adults, diagnosis of ADHD is contingent on self-report, whereas diagnosis in children is supported by information from additional informants (parents and teachers).

- As children enter adolescence and adulthood, symptoms may shift and manifest differently or be less obvious. Symptoms may include:
  - Poor time management
  - Inability to concentrate or focus attention
  - Distractibility
- Other psychiatric disorders present similarly to ADHD but require a very different course of treatment (for example, bipolar disorder).
- Clinicians should assess for possible secondary gains from diagnosis.
- Substance addiction and dependence can disguise or mimic ADHD symptoms.
- Medications used to treat ADHD have a high abuse potential.
- Primary-care clinicians may not be trained in the use of diagnostic or assessment tools to evaluate children and/or adults in whom ADHD is suspected.
- Additional problems may arise, such as medication-induced anxiety, stress, depression, and sleep problems.
- Patient may have difficulty swallowing and unwillingness to eat.
- Patient may have issues with medicating (e.g., self-medicating, not medicating, or over-medicating) (Bahn et al., 2020).

Essential Facts

Adolescents and adults with newly diagnosed ADHD symptoms should be screened for signs of substance use, anxiety, depression, and learning disabilities.

Essential Facts

During childhood, males are more than twice as likely as girls to receive a diagnosis of ADHD.

RISK ASSESSMENT PRACTICE CONSIDERATIONS

- Chromosomal disorders
- Family history (genetics)
- History of central nervous system (CNS) infection
- History of developmental, neurologic, medical, or mental health conditions
- History of trauma
- Low birth weight
- Perinatal stress
- Poverty
- Premature birth
- Prenatal smoking, alcohol, or substance exposure

The following are risk factors for ADHD that require additional research because current data are inconclusive (Bahn et al., 2020; Robberecht et al., 2020):

- Decreased methylation of relevant genes
- Dietary sensitivities
  - Food additives (artificial colors, flavors, and preservatives)
  - Refined sugar
  - Yeast
  - Food sensitivity
  - Vitamin deficiencies (i.e., iron, zinc, magnesium, vitamin D)
- Environmental elements
- Epigenetic
- Interaction of genes and nutrition
- Metal toxicity or neurotoxin exposure
- Mitochondrial dysfunctions
- Oxidative stress

Essential Facts

Reports from twin and adoption studies have consistently shown high heritability of approximately 75% for childhood ADHD (Bahn et al., 2020).

Currently, there are no neuropsychological tests with established diagnostic applications for ADHD (Bahn et al., 2020; Wolraich et al., 2019). Clinicians use standardized clinical rating and self-report checklists, behavior questionnaires, and/or rating scales to gather the information needed to screen, diagnose, and develop a treatment plan. These tools are also used throughout treatment to track symptoms and monitor treatment progress.

PEDIATRIC AND ADOLESCENT SCREENING TOOLS

Clinicians use the following screening tools to assess children and adolescents for ADHD:

- ADHD Rating Scale-IV
- Child Behavior Checklist
- Conners' Rating Scales
  - Conners' Parent Rating Scale–Revised for Parents/Caregivers
  - Conners' Teacher Rating Scale–Revised for Teachers
  - Conners-Wells' Adolescent Self–Report Scale for Teenagers
- National Initiative for Children's Healthcare Quality (NICHQ) Vanderbilt Assessment Scales

- National Initiative for Children's Healthcare Quality (NICHQ)–Vanderbilt Assessment Scale -Parent Informant
- National Initiative for Children's Healthcare Quality (NICHQ) Vanderbilt Assessment Scale - Teacher Informant

ADULT AND OLDER ADULT SCREENING TOOLS

Clinicians use the following screening tools to assess adults and older adults for ADHD:

- ADHD Rating Scale IV with Adult Prompts
- Adult ADHD Clinical Diagnostic Scale v1.2
- Adult ADHD Self-Report Scale (ASRS) v1.1
- ASRS v1.1 Screener
- Brown Attention-Deficit Disorder Symptom Assessment Scale for Adults
- Conners' Adult ADHD Rating Scales
- Young ADHD Questionnaire-Self-Report and Young ADHD Questionnaire-Informant-Report

TARGET TREATMENT GOALS

The development of individualized treatment plans for children should address the child's symptoms of inattention, hyperactivity, and impulsivity, along with the child's academic performance, social interactions, and family function. The treatment plan should also include the methods and target goals for treatment, means of monitoring over time, and specific plans for follow-up monitoring. Effective strategies for the treatment of ADHD include a combined approach of pharmacologic, behavioral, and multimodal methods. It is important that target goals are realistic, attainable, and measurable, and that goals are made with input from parents, children, family members, teachers, employment personnel, and so on.

Essential Facts

In 1937, American psychiatrist Charles Bradley discovered that an amphetamine medication reduced ADHD-like symptoms (Faraone et al., 2021).

MEDICATIONS FOR TREATMENT OF ATTENTION DEFICIT HYPERACTIVITY DISORDER IN PEDIATRIC AND ADULT POPULATIONS

Although medication does not cure ADHD, it can be a highly effective way to treat and manage ADHD symptoms. Medications can also help to improve an individual's overall functioning in school, at home, at work, and in the community. First-line therapy for school-aged children (6 years or older) and adolescents who meet diagnostic criteria for ADHD consists of medication with or without behavioral or psychologic interventions (Wolraich et al., 2019). For children under age 6, medication should be considered if behavioral interventions are not adequate (Wolraich et al., 2019). Treatments using stimulant medication such as methylphenidate and dexamphetamine (or dextroamphetamine), combined with nonstimulant atomoxetine (nonstimulant selective noradrenaline reuptake inhibitors), extended release guanfacine, and extended-release clonidine (an alpha 2A agonists) are available; however, despite the available clinical guidelines, the efficacy and safety of ADHD medications remains controversial (Cortese et al., 2018). The benefits and potential adverse effects of pharmacotherapy treatment should be discussed with patients and caregivers. Notably, clinicians must discuss the association between cardiovascular risks (sudden unexpected death [SUD]) and stimulant medications. If an individual has a personal or family history of cardiac disease, SUD, or unexplained exercise intolerance, a consultation with a referral to a cardiologist should be initiated.

Medications that have not been specifically approved by U.S. the Food and Drug Administration (FDA) for treating ADHD but may be helpful include bupropion (Wellbutrin), modafinil (Provigil or Nuvigil), and tricyclic antidepressants (TCAs) such as desipramine (Norpramin), imipramine (Tofranil), and memantine. An electrocardiogram should be obtained prior to starting a TCA in adults and conducted periodically throughout treatment. Bupropion is an NE DA reuptake inhibitor that has shown to be effective in both adults and adolescents (Budur et al., 2005). Bupropion has been associated with an increased risk of drug-induced seizures; therefore, clinicians must use caution when prescribing bupropion for individuals with preexisting seizure or eating disorders (Budur et al., 2005). Modafinil is a wake-promoting DA reuptake inhibitor, and memantine is an N-methyl-daspartate receptor agonist. Due to their sedative effects, short half-life, tolerability, and accessibility, alpha-2A agonists, particularly clonidine, are occasionally used off label to treat sleep-onset insomnia in children with ADHD.

Although it is important to screen older adults with suspected ADHD because people are living longer and retiring later in life, treatment and management of ADHD in older adults can be challenging. American Geriatrics Society Beers Criteria Update Expert Panel's (2019) list of evidence-based recommendations provided strong evidence that amphetamine, armodafinil, and methylphenidate modafinil may possibly cause more harmful than beneficial outcomes. In older adults, stimulant medications can be overstimulating and cause agitation, especially in individuals with mood dysregulation. Furthermore, stimulants must be used with caution in individuals with heart conditions because stimulant medications can cause arrythmias and increase blood pressure. Additionally, polypharmacy (simultaneously using multiple medications) can be a problem if an individual has other comorbid conditions. A combination of lifestyle, behavioral therapy, and medication management is recommended. Tables 9.3 and 9.4 list CNS stimulants, approved by the FDA for the treatment of ADHD, that contain amphetamine and methylphenidate derivatives. Table 9.5 lists ADHD nonstimulant FDA-approved medications.

Table 9.3

Stimulants, Methylphenidate Formulations

Generic Name (Brand Name)	Dosage Forms	FDA Approval	Clinical Considerations
Methylphenidate HCl (Adhansia XR)	Capsule	*Adults:* ADHD, narcolepsy *Non-FDA Uses:* treatment-resistant depression *Pediatrics:* ADHD (6 years and older)*	Long-acting IR and ER Capsule can be opened and mixed with applesauce.
Methylphenidate HCl (Aptensio XR)	Capsule	*Adults:* ADHD, narcolepsy *Pediatrics:* ADHD (≥6 years)* *Older Adult Considerations:***	Long-acting IR and ER Capsule can be opened and mixed with applesauce.
Serdexmethyl-phenidate and dexmethylphenidate (Azstarys)	Capsule	*Adults:* ADHD up to age 65 *Pediatrics:* ADHD ≥6 years* *Older Adult Considerations:***	Long-acting IR and ER Capsule can be opened and mixed with applesauce.
Methylphenidate HCl (Concerta)	Tablet: Long Acting Immediate Extended Release	*Adults:* ADHD *Non-FDA Uses:* narcolepsy, tx-resistant depression *Pediatrics:* ADHD ≥6 years* *Older Adult Considerations:***	Must be swallowed whole with a liquid. Must not be chewed, divided, cut, or crushed.
Methylphenidate (Daytrana)	Transdermal patch	*Adults:* Approved ≥6 years and adolescents *Pediatrics:* ADHD ≥6 years*	Remove 9 hours after application. Place on a clean, dry area of the hip. Encourage use of administration chart included with each carton of DAYTRANA to monitor patch application and removal time, and method of disposal. Do not store in refrigerator or freezer.

*Monitor children for growth and weight.

**Follow standard adult dosing. Start at the lowest dosage and titrate slowly while monitoring the patient for any side effects; assess prior to use for a history of family or patients with a history cardiac disease, structural cardiac abnormalities or other cardiac conditions.

(continued)

Table 9.3

Stimulants, Methylphenidate Formulations (*continued*)

Generic Name (Brand Name)	Dosage Forms	FDA Approval	Clinical Considerations
Dexmethylphenidate HCl (Focalin)	Tablet	*Adults:* ADHD *Pediatrics:* ADHD ≥6 years*	Short-acting IR Only ER is approved for adult populations.
Dexmethylphenidate HCl (Focalin XR)	Capsule	*Adults:* ADHD *Pediatrics:* ADHD ≥6 years*	Long-acting IR and ER Capsule can be opened and mixed with applesauce.
Methylphenidate HCl (Jornay PM)	Capsule	*Adults:* ADHD *Pediatrics:* ADHD ≥6 years* *Older Adult Considerations:***	Long-acting ER Instruct patients to take in the evening between 6:30 and 9:30 to obtain morning symptom control. Capsule can be opened and mixed with applesauce.
Methylphenidate HCl (Metadate CD)	Capsule	*Adults:* ADHD *Pediatrics:* ADHD ≥6 years* *Older Adult Considerations:***	Both IR and ER beads. 30% of the dose is provided by the IR component and 70% of the dose is provided by the ER component. Capsule can be opened and mixed with applesauce.
Methylphenidate HCl (Metadate ER)	Tablet	*Adults:* ADHD, narcolepsy *Pediatrics:* ADHD ≥6 years* *Older Adult Considerations:***	Long-acting IR and ER
Methylphenidate HCl (Methlyn ER Solution)	Solution	*Adults:* ADHD, narcolepsy *Pediatrics:* ADHD ≥6 years* *Older Adult Considerations:***	Short-acting IR

*Monitor children for growth and weight.

**Follow standard adult dosing. Start at the lowest dosage and titrate slowly while monitoring the patient for any side effects assess prior to use for a history of family or patients with a history cardiac disease, structural cardiac abnormalities or other cardiac conditions.

(*continued*)

Table 9.3

Stimulants, Methylphenidate Formulations (*continued*)

Generic Name (Brand Name)	Dosage Forms	FDA Approval	Clinical Considerations
Methylphenidate (Methylphenidate Chewable)	Chewable Tablets	*Adults:* ADHD, narcolepsy *Pediatrics:* ADHD, narcolepsy ≥6 years* *Older Adult Considerations:* **	Short-acting IR
Methylphenidate HCl (Methylphenidate [Cotempla XR-ODT])	ODT Tablet	*Adults:* ADHD *Pediatrics:* ADHD ≥6 years*	Long-acting IR and ER (25% IR/75% ER)
Methylphenidate HCl (Quillichew ER)	Chewable Tablets	*Adults:* ADHD *Pediatrics:* ADHD ≥6 years* *Older Adult Considerations:***	Long-acting IR and ER (30% IR/70% ER)
Methylphenidate HCl (Quillivant XR)	Solution	*Adults:* ADHD *Pediatrics:* ADHD ≥6 years* *Older Adult Considerations:***	Long-acting IR and ER (20% IR/80% ER)
Methylphenidate HCl (Ritalin IR)	Tablet	*Adults:* ADHD, narcolepsy *Pediatrics:* ADHD ≥6 years* *Older Adult Considerations:***	Short-acting IR
Methylphenidate HCl (Ritalin SR)	Capsule	*Adults:* ADHD, narcolepsy *Pediatrics:* ADHD (6 to 12 years old)* *Older Adult Considerations:***	Long-acting IR and ER May be used in place of immediate release Ritalin tablets. Capsule can be opened and mixed with applesauce.

*Monitor children for growth and weight.
**Follow standard adult dosing. Start at the lowest dosage and titrate slowly while monitoring the patient for any side effects; assess prior to use for a history of family or patients with a history cardiac disease, structural cardiac abnormalities or other cardiac conditions.
ADHD, attention deficit hyperactivity disorder; ER, extended-release; FDA, U.S. Food and Drug Administration; IR, immediate-release.

Table 9.4

Stimulants, Amphetamine Derivatives

Generic Name (Brand Name)	Dosage Forms	FDA Approval	Clinical Considerations
Amphetamine mixed salts/tablets (Adderall XR)	Capsules	*Adults:* ADHD, narcolepsy *Pediatrics:* ADHD ≥3 years and older depending on the medication formulation narcolepsy ≥6 years*	Long-acting ER Capsule can be opened and mixed with applesauce.
Amphetamine/ Dextroamphetamine (Adderall)	Tablets	*Adults:* ADHD, narcolepsy *Pediatrics:* ADHD ≥3 years, narcolepsy ≥6*	Short-acting IR
(Adzenys ER)	Solution	*Adults:* ADHD *Pediatrics:* ADHD ≥6 years*	Long-acting ER
(Adzenys XR-ODT)	ODT Tablets	*Adults:* ADHD *Pediatrics:* ADHD ≥3*	Long-acting ER
Dextroamphetamine (Dexedrine Spansule)	Capsule	*Adults:* Only approved for the pediatric population *Pediatrics:* ADHD ≥6*	Long-acting ER
Amphetamine oral suspension	Solution	*Adults:* ADHD *Pediatric:* ADHD ≥6* *Older Adult Considerations:***	Long-acting ER
(Evekeo)	Tablets	*Adults:* ADHD ≥3, narcolepsy ≥6 *Pediatrics:* ADHD ≥3, narcolepsy ≥6; exogenous obesity short-term treatment ≥12	Short-acting IR
(Dyanavel XR)		ADHD children ages 6-17 years	
(Evekeo ODT)	Tablets	*Adults:* ADHD ≥6 *Pediatrics:* ADHD ≥6*	Short-acting IR
Dextroamphetamine sulfate (Mydayis ER Capsule)	Capsules	*Adults:* ADHD, narcolepsy *Pediatrics:* ADHD (13 years and older)* *Older Adult Considerations:***	Long-acting ER Capsule can be opened and mixed with applesauce.

*Monitor children for growth and weight.
**Follow standard adult dosing. Start at the lowest dosage and titrate slowly while monitoring the patient for any side effects; assess prior to use for a history of family or patients with a history cardiac disease, structural cardiac abnormalities or other cardiac conditions.

(*continued*)

Table 9.4

Stimulants, Amphetamine Derivatives (*continued*)

Generic Name (Brand Name)	Dosage Forms	FDA Approval	Clinical Considerations
Dextroamphetamine sulfate (ProCentra)	Solution	*Adults:* only approved for the pediatric population *Pediatrics:* ADHD ≥3 years, narcolepsy 6 to 17 years*	Short-acting IR
(Vyvanse)	Capsules Chewable Tablets	*Adults:* ADHD, BED *Pediatrics:* ADHD ≥6 years *Older Adult Considerations:***	Long-acting ER Regular tablets may be mixed with yogurt, orange juice, or water.
Dextroamphetamine (Zenzedi)	Tablets	*Adults:* only approved for the pediatric population *Pediatrics:* ADHD ≥3 years, narcolepsy 6 to 17 years*	Short-acting IR

*Monitor children for growth and weight.
**Follow standard adult dosing. Start at the lowest dosage and titrate slowly while monitoring the patient for any side effects; assess prior to use for a history of family or patients with a history cardiac disease, structural cardiac abnormalities or other cardiac conditions.
ADHD, attention deficit hyperactivity disorder; BED, binge eating disorder; ER, extended release; FDA, U.S. Food and Drug Administration; IR, immediate release.

Essential Facts

It is important to note that a failed response to stimulant medications does not necessarily dismiss a diagnosis of ADHD. Approximately 30% of individuals with ADHD do not respond adequately to the stimulant medication due to an undiagnosed comorbid condition, psychosocial stressors, or noncompliance (Budur et al., 2005).

Essential Facts

Depending on the severity of the ADHD, it is recommended that children stay on their ADHD medication full-time without breaks; however, some breaks from stimulant medication or a dosage reduction may be considered for less-demanding times during weekends, holidays, and during the summer.

Table 9.5

FDA-Approved Nonstimulants

Generic Name (Brand Name)	Dosage Forms	FDA Approval	Clinical Considerations
Atomoxetine (Strattera)	Tablets	*Adults:* ADHD *Pediatrics:* ADHD *Older Adult Considerations:***	Monitor BP, heart rate, and cardiac function.
Bupropion (Wellbutrin)	IR, SR, and XL Tablets	*Adults:* MDD, seasonal affective disorder (extended-release formulations), smoking cessation (Zyban) *Non-FDA Uses*: ADHD, depression (with bipolar disorder), obesity, antidepressant-associated sexual dysfunction *Off-Label:* ADHD, neuropathic pain *Pediatrics:* safety in pediatric use has not been established *Off-Label:* ADHD *Older Adult Considerations:* may need to be adjusted based on reduced clearance and metabolism	SL tablets should not exceed 200 mg in one dose. XL tablets should not exceed 450 mg in one dose.
Clonidine (Kapvay)	Tablets: ER Tablets ER Patch Injectable Solution	*Adults:* Hypertension, *Off-Label:* acute hypertension, EtOH withdrawal, smoking cessation, restless legs syndrome, Tourette' syndrome, cyclosporine nephrotoxicity, menopausal flushing, dysmenorrhea, opioid withdrawal, post-herpetic neuralgia, psychosis, pheochromocytoma diagnosis *Pediatrics:* ADHD, hypertension, cancer pain; only approved for ages 6 to 17 *Older Adult Considerations:* avoid use in older adults due to risk for orthostatic hypotension and adverse CNS effects	Monitor BP, heart rate, and cardiac function.

*Monitor children for growth and weight.
**Follow standard adult dosing. Start at the lowest dosage and titrate slowly while monitoring the patient for any side effects; assess prior to use for a history of family or patients with a history cardiac disease, structural cardiac abnormalities or other cardiac conditions.

(*continued*)

Table 9.5

FDA-Approved Nonstimulants (*continued*)

Generic Name (Brand Name)	Dosage Forms	FDA Approval	Clinical Considerations
Guanfacine (Intuniv)	Tablets	*Adults:* hypertension *Off-Label:* heroin withdrawal, migraine prophylaxis *Pediatrics:* ADHD *Older Adult Considerations:***	Avoid use in older adults due to risk for orthostatic hypotension and adverse CNS effects.
Viloxazine (Qelbree)	Tablets	*Adults:* only approved for the pediatric population *Pediatrics:* ADHD 12 to 17 years*	Capsule can be opened and mixed with applesauce.

*Monitor children for growth and weight.
**Follow standard adult dosing. Start at the lowest dosage and titrate slowly while monitoring the patient for any side effects; assess prior to use for a history of family or patients with a history cardiac disease, structural cardiac abnormalities or other cardiac conditions.
ADHD, attention deficit hyperactivity disorder; BP, blood pressure; CNS, central nervous system; ER, extended release; EtOH, ethyl alcohol; FDA, U.S. Food and Drug Administration; IR, immediate release; MDD, major depressive disorder; SR, sustained release; XL, extended release.

Essential Facts

Neuropsychological testing alone does not provide an accurate diagnosis of ADHD.

CRITERIA FOR INITIATING STIMULANT AND NONSTIMULANT ATTENTION DEFICIT HYPERACTIVITY DISORDER MEDICATIONS

- ADHD diagnosis is documented and confirmed based on *DSM-5* criteria.
- Arrangements are made with school to administer medication if indicated.
- Consult with specialists if comorbid conditions are present.
- Ensure there is no concern of substance misuse in the home.
- Ensure there is no history of substantial anxiety.
- Ensure there is no known prior seizure disorder or risk.
- Ensure there is no prior sensitivity or reaction to medication.
- Ensure there is normal blood pressure.
- Ensure there is normal heart rate.

Essential Facts

According to Groenman et al. (2013), individuals with ADHD who received psychostimulant treatment had a lower risk of developing substance-use disorders than those who did not receive the treatment.

Essential Facts

Individuals with preexisting psychosis, agitation, or a history of drug abuse should be carefully monitored when using ADHD medication.

PSYCHOSTIMULANTS

Mechanism of Action

Therapeutic action of methylphenidate and amphetamine involves the dopaminergic and noradrenergic neurotransmitter systems in prefrontal and striatal regions and increases in DA and NE concentrations in the PFC. Methylphenidate and amphetamine derivatives stimulate the cerebral cortex and subcortical brain structures and block the reuptake of NE and DA into presynaptic neurons (Yoo et al., 2020). Stimulants are the first-line pharmacologic treatment for both children and adults with ADHD. It is important to consider the variations in medication delivery technologies that have been developed to address individual patient needs.

NONSTIMULANTS

Alpha$_2$-Adrenergic Agonist Mechanism of Action

Alpha$_2$-adrenergic agonists improve PFC functioning by stimulating postsynaptic alpha-2A adrenergic receptors, so they inhibit the production of cyclic adenosine monophosphate and close hyperpolarization-activated cyclic nucleotide-gated channels, thus enhancing the effectiveness of the signal of the pyramidal neurons of the PFC (Sallee, 2010). Alpha2-adrenergic agonists improve cognitive performance by mimicking norepinephrine effects at the alpha 2A adrenoreceptors in the PFC. Because of their prominent alpha-2B receptor activity, alpha$_2$-adrenergic agonists (guanfacine and clonidine) are frequently used adjunctively as soporifics to help with stimulant-induced sleep disturbances such as delay in sleep onset, resistance to going to bed, wakefulness, restlessness, and so on.

Alpha2-Adrenergic Agonists

- Intuniv (Tenex, guanfacine extended release)
  - 6 to 12 years: 1 to 4 mg; starting dose (SD): 1 mg; 13 to 17 years: 1 to 7 mg; SD: 1 mg weight-based dosing: SD: 0.05 to 0.08 mg/kg/day; may increase to 0.12 mg/kg/day
- Kapvay (Catapres, clonidine extended release)
  - 6 to 17 years: 0.1 to 0.2 mg BID; starting dose: 0.1 mg qHS

SELECTIVE NOREPINEPHRINE REUPTAKE INHIBITOR MECHANISM OF ACTION

Atomoxetine increases NE and DA within the PFC, but not in the nucleus accumbens or striatum. This increase is beneficial in the treatment of ADHD because DA activation in the subcortical nucleus accumbens and striatum is associated with many stimulant-associated side effects and an increase in abuse potential (Callahan et al., 2019).

Essential Facts

Atomoxetine Has No Abuse Potential

First-line therapy for children and adults at risk for substance use disorders may be preferred over stimulants, especially in individuals with comorbid anxiety disorders.

Selective Norepinephrine Reuptake

- Strattera (atomoxetine)
  - less than 70 kg: 0.5 mg/kg x greater than 3d, then 1.2 mg/kg (max: 1.4 mg/kg, not to exceed 100 mg); greater than 70 kg: 40 mg/kg x greater than 3d, then 80 mg (max: 100 mg)
- Qelbree (viloxazine)
  - 6 to 11 years: 100 to 400 mg; SD: 100 mg; 12 to 17 years: 200 to 400 mg; starting dose: 200 mg

PRESCRIBING CONSIDERATIONS

Pharmacologic treatment in conjunction with behavioral interventions is the optimal treatment option to improve excessive physical activity, inattention, impulsivity and poor self-control, physical and verbal aggression, and low academic productivity in individuals with ADHD. When initiating pharmacotherapy, the rule of thumb is to start low and go slow. For children who require medication during the school day, it is important to develop a plan to ensure that medication is administered in accordance with the child's individualized education plan. Additional considerations to include when weighing the advantages of one drug over another are safety, tolerability, effectiveness, price, and simplicity, also referred to as the STEPS framework of prescribing (Shaughnessy, 2003). Clinicians should also consider the following factors when prescribing medication:

- Concurrent medications
- Duration of action (long acting/extended release, immediate release, combined treatment)
- Form of medication (liquid, capsule, tablet, dissolvable tablet, chewable, sprinkle, patch)
- Insurance coverage
- Past response to medication
- Patient preference
- Side-effects profile

Essential Facts

STEPS framework in medication prescribing:

- Safety
- Tolerability
- Effectiveness
- Price
- Simplicity

Essential Facts

The nonstimulant NE/DA reuptake inhibitor bupropion (used for the treatment of depression and for smoking cessation) has also been shown to be effective in the treatment of ADHD (Verbeeck et al., 2017).

Side Effects Experienced With Psychostimulants

- "Black Box" warning for suicidal thoughts
- Cardiovascular (tachycardia)

- Constipation
- Dry mouth
- Erectile dysfunction
- Gastrointestinal upset
- Hand tremor
- Headaches
- High potential for abuse and dependence
- Insomnia, daytime sleepiness
- Nervousness
- Priapism
- Psychosis/mania
- "Rebound" irritability
- Slowed growth
- Tic disorders
- Weight loss, anorexia

Side Effects Experienced With Nonstimulant Medications

The following side effects may be experienced when taking clonidine and guanfacine:

- Changes in appetite and weight; constipation; depression; dizziness; drowsiness; dry mouth/thirst; fainting; fatigue; heart rate drop; hypotension/postural dizziness; irritability; itching; and rebound hypertension

The following side effects may be experienced with atomoxetine (Strattera):

- Headaches; increased blood pressure; increased heart rate; mild appetite suppression/weight loss; nausea; sexual dysfunction in older adolescents/ young adults; tiredness; upset stomach; vomiting
- Black Box warning for suicidal thoughts
- Dose adjustment with CYP2D6 inhibitors

The following side effects may be experienced with bupropion (Wellbutrin), an off-label medication used to treat ADHD that has not been approved by the FDA:

- Anxiety; dry mouth; increased energy; irregular heartbeat; irritability; mania; restlessness; risk of drug-induced seizures (caution for individuals with preexisting seizure, substance use or eating disorders); skin rash, hives, or itching
- Black Box warning for suicidal thoughts and/or actions in children and adults

Essential Facts

Atomoxetine is useful in patients with ADHD who have a comorbid substance abuse disorder or tic disorder.

Essential Facts

The FDA has added a Black Box warning to the package insert for stimulants and atomoxetine. The warning suggests that some children may experience suicidal thoughts after starting this medication. Atomoxetine also may increase heart rate and blood pressure.

Essential Facts

Behavioral rebound is a change in behavior that occurs in some individuals when the stimulant medication is wearing off. Symptoms may include irritableness, increase in overactivity, impulsivity, and inattention in the late afternoon or evening.

BEHAVIORIAL THERAPY

Psychosocial and behavioral techniques can be applied in a variety of settings, including school, home, work, and community settings. Psychosocial interventions and behavioral interventions can help individuals with ADHD gain social skills and have more positive and satisfying interactions with peers and family members. Therapy can also help individuals recognize visual and audio cues, achieve academic and occupational success, manage self-esteem issues, and develop structure and/or routines.

MAINTENANCE PHASE OF TREATMENT

At follow-up appointments, the nurse practitioner should discuss (a) medication compliance, (b) possible adverse drug effects, (c) sleep duration and quality, and (d) experiences with hobbies, athletics, peer activities, family interactions, and academic or occupational performance. Practitioners should also monitor the patient's weight, body mass index, and growth using standardized charts. Medication effects can also be monitored by reviewing ADHD-specific rating scales, and medication adjustments can be made accordingly.

ONGOING MONITORING

- Alcohol and substance use
- Caffeine intake
- Laboratory tests when indicated
- Medication compliance
- Mood swings
- Signs of mania or psychosis
- Sleep patterns, sleep changes, and sleep hygiene
- Social, academic, occupational functioning decline
- Suicide assessment

- Surveillance for possible comorbidities
- Violence and self-harmful behaviors
- Weight changes

CRITERIA FOR REFERRAL

Most primary-care providers can manage treatment for children who have ADHD and no complex comorbidities. Individuals with (a) comorbid developmental abnormalities, (b) psychiatric conditions that do not respond to pharmacotherapy, (c) concurrent intellectual or developmental disorders, (d) learning disabilities, (e) visual or hearing impairments, (f) abuse history, (g) a tendency toward severe aggression levels, (h) seizure disorders, and (i) coexisting learning and/or emotional problems should be referred to a psychiatrist, pediatric neurologist, education specialist, psycho-pharmacologist, or developmental, clinical, or behavioral specialist (Tran, 2021). Additionally, referrals are necessary for those who have extreme difficulties in their relationships with peers, teachers, family, or workplace. Timely referrals are essential to support accurate diagnosis and help ensure that the plan of care for the child or adolescent is individualized. Individualized treatment plans help optimize the patient outcomes, improve quality of life and well-being, and alleviate current and potential dysfunctions of daily living (Tran, 2021). Children and adolescents with ADHD may also benefit from psychosocial treatments such as behavioral therapy and training interventions (Wolraich et al., 2019).

SUMMARY

ADHD is a multifaceted developmental disorder that impacts individuals, families, and educators. ADHD has been associated with reduced academic and occupational achievement due to cognitive and motivational difficulties and decreased social functioning. Despite increased guidelines for the assessment and treatment of ADHD, optimal routine care within outpatient treatment settings remains unknown. Clinicians must have the necessary knowledge and skills to accurately diagnose ADHD and competently manage this disorder to optimize patient outcomes (Tran, 2021).

RESOURCES

It is important to provide education to patients and family members through various resources, including websites, books, pamphlets, and so on. The following is a list of resources for ADHD education and management:

- Children and Adults with Attention Deficit/Hyperactivity Disorder (CHADD): www.chadd.org
- Centers for Disease Control and Prevention (CDC): Attention-Deficit/Hyperactivity Disorder (ADHD): www.cdc.gov/ncbddd/adhd
- American Academy of Pediatrics (AAP): Clinical report on promoting optimal development—Identifying infants and young children with developmental disorders through developmental surveillance and screening

- ADHD International Consensus Statement (World ADHD Federation): www.adhd-federation.org/publications/international-consensus-statement.html
- European Consensus by the European Network of Adult ADH: www.eunetworkadultadhd.com
- Canadian Attention Deficit Hyperactivity Disorder Resource Alliance (CADDRA): www.caddra.ca
- The American Academy of Child and Adolescent Psychiatry (AACAP): www.aacap.org/AACAP/Families_and_Youth/Facts_for_Families/FFF-Guide/Children-Who-Cant-Pay-Attention-Attention-Deficit-Hyperactivity-Disorder-006.aspx
- Choosing Wisely: Do not order a screening EKG prior to initiation of attention-deficit/hyperactivity disorder (ADHD) therapy in asymptomatic, otherwise healthy pediatric patients with no personal or family history of cardiac disease
- Society for Developmental and Behavioral Pediatrics (SDBP): Clinical practice guideline for the assessment and treatment of children and adolescents with complex attention-deficit/hyperactivity disorder
- AAP: Clinical practice guideline for the diagnosis, evaluation, and treatment of attention-deficit/hyperactivity disorder in children and adolescents
- AAP: Clinical report on school-aged children who are not progressing academically—Considerations for pediatricians
- National Attention Deficit Disorder Association (ADDA): www.add.org

REVIEW QUESTIONS

1. A timely referral to a clinical or behavioral specialist is indicated for which one of the following?
   a. Children with comorbid developmental abnormalities, abuse history, a tendency toward severe aggression levels, and coexisting learning and/or emotional problems
   b. Children who do not achieve an adequate response to attention deficit hyperactivity disorder (ADHD) pharmacotherapy
   c. Children who have visual or hearing impairments or seizure disorders with ADHD symptoms
   d. All of the above warrant a referral to a specialist.
2. Which one of the following is the area of the brain that regulates attention by sustaining focus while reducing distractibility (i.e., the area most affected in patients with attention deficit hyperactivity disorder [ADHD])?
   a. The prefrontal cortex (PFC)
   b. The amygdala
   c. The cerebellum
   d. The hippocampus
3. Which one of the following statements is not true regarding risk factors for attention deficit hyperactivity disorder (ADHD)?
   a. Heredity makes a large contribution to the expression of ADHD.
   b. Prenatal exposure to alcohol and tobacco, premature delivery, and significantly low birth weight have all been found to contribute to the risk for ADHD.

c. High lead levels have been shown to increase the risk for ADHD.
d. It has been absolutely determined that ADHD risk factors include excessive sugar intake, excessive television viewing, or poor parenting management.

4. As part of the attention deficit hyperactivity disorder (ADHD) evaluation, a comprehensive evaluation includes which one of the following?
   a. An intelligence quotient (IQ) test
   b. Gathering information from multiple sources, which can include ADHD symptom checklists, standardized behavior rating scales, a detailed history of past and current functioning, and information obtained from collateral sources
   c. An MRI
   d. An electroencephalography (EEG) to measure the brain's overall neuronal activity
5. Which answer choice below is not a symptom of ADHD?
   a. Impulsivity
   b. Fidgeting
   c. Stuttering
   d. Inattention

REFERENCES

American Geriatrics Society Beers Criteria® Update Expert Panel. (2019). American Geriatrics Society 2019 Updated AGS Beers Criteria® for potentially inappropriate medication use in older adults. *Journal of the American Geriatrics Society, 67*(4), 674–694. https://doi.org/10.1111/jgs.15767

American Psychiatric Association. (2013). *Diagnostic and statistical manual of mental disorders* (5th ed.). https://doi.org/10.1176/appi.books.9780890425596

Bahn, G. H., Lee, Y. S., Yoo, H. K., Kim, E. J., Park, S., Han, D. H., Hong, M., Kim, B., Lee, S. I., Bhang, S. Y., Lee, S. Y., Hong, J. P., & Joung, Y. S. (2020). Development of the Korean practice parameter for adult attention-deficit/hyperactivity disorder. *Journal of Child & Adolescent Psychiatry, 31*(1), 5–25. https://doi.org/10.5765/jkacap.190030

Budur, K., Mathews, M., Adetunji, B., Mathews, M., & Mahmud, J. (2005). Non-stimulant treatment for attention deficit hyperactivity disorder. *Psychiatry, 2*(7), 44–48. https://www.ncbi.nlm.nih.gov/pmc/articles/PMC3000197

Callahan, P. M., Plagenhoef, M. R., Blake, D. T., & Terry, A. V. (2019). Atomoxetine improves memory and other components of executive function in young-adult rats and aged rhesus monkeys. *Neuropharmacology, 155*, 65–75. https://doi.org/10.1016/j.neuropharm.2019.05.016

Children and Adults with Attention-Deficit/Hyperactivity Disorder. (n.d.). More older adults receiving a new ADHD diagnosis. Retrieved September 4, 2021, from https://chadd.org/adhd-news/adhd-news-adults/more-older-adults-receiving-a-new-adhd-diagnosis

Cortese, S., Adamo, N., Del Giovane, C., Mohr-Jensen, C., Hayes, A. J., Carucci, S., Atkinson, L. Z., Tessari, L., Banaschewski, T., Coghill, D., Hollis, C., Simonoff, E., Zuddas, A., Barbui, C., Purgato, M., Steinhausen, H. C., Shokraneh, F., Xia, J., & Cipriani, A. (2018). Comparative efficacy and tolerability of medications for attention-deficit hyperactivity disorder in children, adolescents, and adults: A systematic review and network meta-analysis. *Lancet Psychiatry, 5*(9), 727–738. https://doi.org/10.1016/S2215-0366(18)30269-4

Faraone, S. V., Banaschewski, T., Coghill, D., Zheng, Y., Biederman, J., Bellgrove, M. A., Newcorn, J. H., Gignac, M., Al Saud, N. M., Manor, I., Rohde, L. A., Yang, L., Cortese, S., Almagor, D., Stein, M. A., Albatti, T. H., Aljoudi, H. F., Alqahtani, M., Asherson, P., … Wang, Y. (2021). The World Federation of ADHD International Consensus Statement: 208 evidence-based conclusions about the disorder. *Neuroscience and Biobehavioral Reviews, 128*, 789–818. https://doi.org/10.1016/j.neubiorev.2021.01.022

Faraone, S. V., Silverstein, M. J., Antshel, K., Biederman, J., Goodman, D. W., Mason, O., Nierenberg, A. A., Rostain, A., Stein, M. A., & Adler, L. A. (2019). The adult ADHD quality measures initiative. *Journal of Attention Disorders, 23*(10), 1063–1078. https://doi.org/10.1177/1087054718804354

Franke, B., Michelini, G., Asherson, P., Banaschewski, T., Bilbow, A., Buitelaar, J. K., Cormand, B., Faraone, S. V., Ginsberg, Y., Haavik, J., Kuntsi, J., Larsson, H., Lesch, K. P., Ramos-Quiroga, J. A., Réthelyi, J. M., Ribases, M., & Reif, A. (2018). Live fast, die young? A review on the developmental trajectories of ADHD across the lifespan. *European Neuropsychopharmacology, 28*(10), 1059–1088. https://doi.org/10.1016/j.euroneuro.2018.08.001

Groenman, A., Oosterlaan, J., Rommelse, N., Franke, B., Greven, C., Hoekstra, P., Hartman, C. A., Luman, M., Roeyers, H., Oades, R. D., Sargeant, J. A., Buitelaar, J. K., & Faraone, S. (2013). Stimulant treatment for attention-deficit hyperactivity disorder and risk of developing substance use disorder. *British Journal of Psychiatry, 203*(2), 112–119. https://doi.org/10.1192/bjp.bp.112.124784

Holbrook, J. R., Cuffe, S. P., Cai, B., Visser, S. N., Forthofer, M. S., Bottai, M., Ortaglia, A., & McKeown, R. E. (2016). Persistence of parent-reported ADHD symptoms from childhood through adolescence in a community sample. *Journal of Attention Disorders, 20*(1), 11–20. https://doi.org/10.1177/1087054714539997

Katusic, M. Z., Voigt, R. G., Colligan, R. C., Weaver, A. L., Homan, K. J., & Barbaresi, W. J. (2011). Attention-deficit hyperactivity disorder in children with high intelligence quotient: results from a population-based study. *Journal of Developmental and Behavioral Pediatrics*, 32(2), 103–109. https://doi.org/10.1097/DBP.0b013e318206d700

Katzman, M. A., Bilkey, T. S., Chokka, P. R., Fallu, A., & Klassen, L. J. (2017). Adult ADHD and comorbid disorders: Clinical implications of a dimensional approach. *BMC Psychiatry, 17*(1), Article 302. https://doi.org/10.1186/s12888-017-1463-3

Klein, M., Onnink, M., van Donkelaar, M., Wolfers, T., Harich, B., Shi, Y., Dammers, J., Arias-Vásquez, A., Hoogman, M., & Franke, B. (2017). Brain imaging genetics in ADHD and beyond – Mapping pathways from gene to disorder at different levels of complexity. *Neuroscience and Biobehavioral Reviews, 80*, 115–155. https://doi.org/10.1016/j.neubiorev.2017.01.013

Morris-Rosendahl, D. J., & Crocq, M. A. (2020). Neurodevelopmental disorders—the history and future of a diagnostic concept. *Dialogues in Clinical Neuroscience, 22*(1), 65–72. https://doi.org/10.31887/DCNS.2020.22.1/macrocq

Robberecht, H., Verlaet, A., Breynaert, A., De Bruyne, T., & Hermans, N. (2020). Magnesium, iron, zinc, copper and selenium status in attention-deficit/hyperactivity disorder (ADHD). *Molecules, 25*(19), Article 4440. https://doi.org/10.3390/molecules25194440

Rosenblum, S., Zandani, I. E., Deutsch-Castel, T., & Meyer, S. (2019). The Child Evaluation Checklist (CHECK): A screening questionnaire for detecting daily functional "red flags" of underrecognized neurodevelopmental disorders among preschool children. *Occupational Therapy International*, 2019, Article 6891831. https://doi.org/10.1155/2019/6891831

Sallee, F. R. (2010). The role of alpha2-adrenergic agonists in attention-deficit/hyperactivity disorder. *Postgraduate Medicine*, *122*(5), 78–87. https://doi.org/10.3810/pgm.2010.09.2204

Savatt, J. M., & Myers, S. M. (2021). Genetic testing in neurodevelopmental disorders. *Frontiers in Pediatrics*, *9*, Article 526779. https://doi.org/10.3389/fped.2021.526779

Shaughnessy, A. F. (2003). STEPS drug updates. *American Family Physician*, *68*(12), 2342–2348. https://www.aafp.org/pubs/afp/issues/2003/1215/p2342.html

Solanto, M. V. (2000). The predominantly inattentive subtype of attention-deficit/hyperactivity disorder. *CNS Spectrums*, *5*(6), 45–51. https://doi.org/10.1017/s1092852900007069

Storebø, O. J., Pedersen, N., Ramstad, E., Kielsholm, M. L., Nielsen, S. S., Krogh, H. B., Moreira-Maia, C. R., Magnusson, F. L., Holmskov, M., Gerner, T., Skoog, M., Rosendal, S., Groth, C., Gillies, D., Buch Rasmussen, K., Gauci, D., Zwi, M., Kirubakaran, R., Håkonsen, S. J., … Gluud, C. (2018). Methylphenidate for attention deficit hyperactivity disorder (ADHD) in children and adolescents – Assessment of adverse events in non-randomised studies. *Cochrane Database of Systematic Reviews*, *5*(5), Article CD012069. https://doi.org/10.1002/14651858.CD012069

Tetering, M., Laan, A., Kogel, C. H., Groot, R., & Jolles, J. (2020). Sex differences in self-regulation in early, middle and late adolescence: A large-scale cross-sectional study. *PloS One*, *15*(1), Article e0227607. https://doi.org/10.1371/journal.pone.0227607

Tran, T. (2021). Diagnosis of attention deficit/hyperactivity disorder in children and adolescents: A helpful guide. *Pediatric Nursing*, *47*(4), 202–207.

Verbeeck, W., Bekkering, G. E., Van den Noortgate, W., & Kramers, C. (2017). Bupropion for attention deficit hyperactivity disorder (ADHD) in adults. *Cochrane Database of Systematic Reviews*, *10*(10), Article CD009504. https://doi.org/10.1002/14651858.CD009504.pub2

Wolraich, M. L., Hagan, J. F., Jr, Allan, C., Chan, E., Davison, D., Earls, M., Evans, S. W., Flinn, S. K., Froehlich, T., Frost, J., Holbrook, J. R., Lehmann, C. U., Lessin, H. R., Okechukwu, K., Pierce, K. L., Winner, J. D., Zurhellen, W. (2019). Clinical practice guideline for the diagnosis, evaluation, and treatment of attention-deficit/hyperactivity disorder in children and adolescents. *Pediatrics*, *144*(4), Article e20192528. https://doi.org/10.1542/peds.2019-2528

Xing, B., Li, Y.-C., & Gao, W.-J. (2016). Norepinephrine versus dopamine and their interaction in modulating synaptic function in the prefrontal cortex. *Brain Research*, *1641*(Pt. B), 217–233. https://doi.org/10.1016/j.brainres.2016.01.005

Yoo, J. H., Sharma, V., Kim, J.-W., McMakin, D. L., Hong, S.-B., Zalesky, A., Kim, B.-N., & Ryan, N. D. (2020). Prediction of sleep side effects following methylphenidate treatment in ADHD youth. *NeuroImage: Clinical*, *26*, Article 102030. https://doi.org/10.1016/j.nicl.2019.102030

10

Antidementia

Neurocognitive disorders (NCDs), previously referred to as dementia, are syndromes that affect the brain. NCDs are characterized by a progressive decline in cognitive functioning that involves loss of memory, difficulty thinking, and changes in mood and behavior. The term "dementia" is still used to describe degenerative dementia that affects older adults. The term "cognition" refers to the process of receiving knowledge and understanding in areas such as psychomotor speed, attention, working memory, declarative memory (verbal and visual), and executive functioning, including planning, decision-making, response inhibition, and cognitive flexibility (Chakrabarty et al., 2016).

In this chapter you will learn:

1. How to identify the common presentations of neurocognitive disorders (NCDs)
2. How to apply the assessment principles of NCDs
3. How to identify screening tools for NCDs
4. How to compare pharmacologic options and deliver pharmacologic interventions when needed
5. How to apply the management principles for dementia
6. How to consider medication safety in the treatment of NCDs

According to the *Diagnostic and Statistical Manual of Mental Disorders* (5th ed.; *DSM-5*; American Psychiatric Association [APA], 2013), neurocognitive disorders (NCDs) possess distinct criteria and are categorized into three subcategories: (a) delirium, (b) mild NCD, and (c) major NCD (Sachdev et al., 2015). Subtypes of mild NCDs and major NCDs include Alzheimer's disease (AD), vascular disease, frontotemporal lobar degeneration, cortical Lewy body disease, traumatic brain injury, substance/medication use, human immunodeficiency virus (HIV) infection, Prion disease, Parkinson's disease, Huntington's disease, major or mild neurocognitive disorder due to another medical condition, multiple etiologies, or unspecified (APA, 2013).

NCDs involve loss of memory, difficulty thinking, disorientation, and changes in mood and behavior that impact an individual's functioning and independence. The hallmark symptoms for major NCDs include a decline in one or more of the following cognitive domains: (a) learning and memory, (b) executive function, (c) language, (d) complex attention, (e) perceptual–motor, and (f) social cognition. Individuals with major NCDs also experience loss of independence in managing everyday activities as a result of their functional impairment (APA, 2013; Sachdev et al., 2015).

AD, vascular dementia, and Lewy body dementia are common neurocognitive conditions that affect older adults (Raulin et al., 2019). AD is a progressive condition found in approximately 70% of autopsies of people with dementia, and approximately 1% to 2% of individuals live with AD by the age of 65. This percentage doubles every 5 years until at least the age of 90 (McShane et al., 2019). In 2015, the World Health Organization (WHO) estimated the number of people living with dementia at 35.6 million, with this number expected to double by 2030 and triple by 2050 (as cited in Piers et al., 2018).

Although the cause of AD and its pathogenesis are unknown, the presence of the ε4 allele of apolipoprotein E (APOE) is one of the strongest genetic risk factors for the development of late-onset AD and is present in approximately 17% to 30% of individuals with AD (McShane et al., 2019; Raulin et al., 2019; Williams et al., 2020). According to Williams et al. (2020), individuals with AD with the APOE4 isoform have accelerated onset of dementia, worsened memory functioning, and a higher amyloid β (Aβ) plaque burden than those who are not APOE4 carriers (James & Bennett, 2019). APOE is a lipoprotein involved in various cellular brain functions, such as neuronal signaling, neuroinflammation, and glucose metabolism. Cerebrovascular dementia occurs when blood vessels in the brain are damaged, usually due to infarction(s), atherosclerosis, arteriolosclerosis, and white matter changes (James & Bennett, 2019). Lewy body dementia has been associated with an abnormal accumulation of the synaptic protein alpha-synuclein, which has also been found in patients with AD and Parkinson's disease (Henderson et al., 2019). According to James and Bennett (2019), older persons diagnosed with AD at autopsy also have vascular pathologies; therefore, mixed pathologies in the diagnosis of AD are not uncommon, with its prevalence increasing with age.

Essential Facts

AD is the most common type of dementia. By age 65, approximately one or two people out of 100 have AD, with the rate doubling every 5 years (McShane et al., 2019).

Essential Facts

What is now referred to as NCDs in the *DSM-5* was previously referred to as "Delirium, Dementia, and Amnestic and Other Cognitive Disorders" in the *DSM-IV* (Sachdev et al., 2015, pp. 8–9).

Essential Facts

The brain circuits involving the prefrontal cortex, parietal cortex, basal ganglia, thalamus, hippocampus, and amygdala are responsible for cognitive processes.

As the population ages, the overall burden of dementia is increasing worldwide. Globally, an estimated 50,000,000 people live with dementia, and this number is estimated to increase to 152,000,000 by 2050 (GBD 2016 Dementia Collaborators, 2019). Dementia affects individuals, their families, and the economy. In primary care, approximately 70% to 80% of individuals diagnosed with dementia have other chronic comorbid conditions (Livingston et al., 2020). Annual global costs for dementia-related expenses are estimated at $1,000,000,000,000 due to multimorbidity challenges, such as difficulties with managing healthcare services, increases in hospitalization rates, and rapid functional decline rates (Livingston et al., 2020).

DIAGNOSTIC CRITERIA FOR DEMENTIA

The following list represents the clinical features of neurocognitive dementia:

- Apraxia
- Behavioral and psychologic symptoms
- Impairment to executive function and judgment/problem-solving
- Impairments in other cognitive domains
- Memory impairment
- Motor signs
- Olfactory dysfunction
- Seizures
- Sleep disturbances

In primary-care settings, embedding screening questions regarding subjective memory complaints can be useful first steps to identify cognitive changes during early stages. Tables 10.1 through 10.3 discuss the domains included in the Mini Mental State Examination (MMSE), key features of

Table 10.1

The Mini Mental State Examination Scoring

Severity	Symptoms and/or Action Steps
Mild AD: MMSE score of 20 or higher	Combination of loss of memory, disorientation, and loss of insight
Moderate AD: MMSE score of 10–20	Marked impairments to manage everyday tasks
Severe dementia: MMSE score of 10 or less	Profound functioning impairments Twenty-four-hour supervision is required

AD, Alzheimer's disease; MMSE, Mini Mental State Examination

Table 10.2

Key Features of Neurodevelopmental Disorders

Disorder	Key Features
Delirium ▪ Substance intoxication delirium ▪ Substance withdrawal delirium ▪ Medication-induced delirium ▪ Delirium due to another medical condition ▪ Delirium due to multiple etiologies ▪ Other specified delirium ▪ Unspecified delirium	▪ Acute onset (hours to a few days) of mental status abnormalities ▪ Rapid onset and fluctuations of symptoms ▪ Disturbance in attention or reduced ability to focus, sustain, and shift attention, and reduced orientation to the environment ▪ Cognitive deficits (memory, perception, and language impairments; disorientation; inattention, altered level of consciousness; and language, visuospatial ability, or perception impairments) ▪ A medical condition or substance caused the disturbance
Major and mild NCDs ▪ Major NCD ▪ Mild NCD ▪ Major or mild NCD due to AD ▪ Major or mild frontotemporal NCD ▪ Major or mild NCD with Lewy bodies ▪ Major or mild vascular NCD ▪ Major or mild NCD due to traumatic brain injury ▪ Substance/medication-induced major or mild NCD ▪ Major or mild NCD due to HIV infection ▪ Major or mild NCD due to prior disease ▪ Major or mild NCD due to Parkinson's disease ▪ Major or mild NCD due to Huntington's disease	An acquired disorder associated with cognitive decline in one or more domains: ▪ Learning and memory ▪ Executive function ▪ Language ▪ Complex attention ▪ Perceptual motor ▪ Social cognition ▪ Mild NCD differs from major NCD by severity of the cognitive deficits and impact of functional impairment on independence and everyday activities ▪ Individuals with mild NCD can manage their deficits with compensatory strategies

(*continued*)

Table 10.2

Key Features of Neurodevelopmental Disorders (*continued*)

Disorder	Key Features
Major or mild NCD due to another medical condition Major or mild NCD due to multiple etiologies	Exclusions for diagnosis: ▪ Presence of delirium ▪ Another mental disorder responsible for cognitive deficit
Unspecified NCD	

AD, Alzheimer's disease; NCD, neurocognitive disorder

Table 10.3

Parkinson's Disease Dementia Versus Dementia With Lewy Bodies

Parkinson's Disease Dementia	Lewy Bodies Dementia
Individuals have had parkinsonism a year or more before developing dementia-related symptoms.	Onset of dementia symptoms and parkinsonism symptoms are closer in time.

NCDs, and the major clinical distinction between Parkinson's disease dementia and dementia with Lewy bodies.

DIFFERENTIAL DIAGNOSIS

Since there is no single behavioral marker that reliably discriminates AD from the other dementias, it is important to consider other underlying pathology in patients with cognitive complaints, such as vascular conditions and other neurodegenerative conditions, including the following:

- AD
- Alcohol-related dementia
- Creutzfeld–Jacob disease
- Delirium
- Degenerative diseases, including age-related cognitive decline, Huntington's Chorea disease, Parkinson's disease, and Pick disease
- Depression, anxiety
- Frontotemporal dementia
- Heavy-metal poisoning (lead poisoning)
- Hormonal imbalance
- Infectious disease (HIV or acquired immunodeficiency syndrome, Creutzfeldt–Jakob disease, meningitis, encephalitis, or syphilis)
- Lewy body dementia
- Nutritional deficiency (vitamin B_{12} deficiency)
- Parkinson dementia

Table 10.4

Risk Factors for Dementia

Areas of Risk	Specific Risk Factors
Genetic factors	Having a first-degree relative with AD (this is the greatest risk factor for developing AD) Possessing the *APOE4* gene; increased risk in females
Medical risk factors	Diabetes, hypertension, elevated cholesterol, cerebral injury (trauma or stroke), hearing impairment, kidney disease, liver disease, and thyroid disorder
Sociodemographic risk factors	Lower educational attainment, low levels of physical activity, low participation in cognitive activities, low social contact or leisure activities, poor diet and nutrition (obesity), poor sleep, air pollution
Psychologic risk factors	Depression, smoking, excessive alcohol consumption

AD, Alzheimer's disease

Table 10.4 provides patient risk factors associated with dementia.

Essential Facts

Exercise may reduce risks of developing diseases of the circulatory system associated with inactivity, thus lowering the risk of vascular dementia.

Essential Facts

Reading, doing puzzles, playing games, and other cognitively stimulating exercises are associated with a lower risk for AD.

Essential Facts

General practitioners fail to identify about 50% of mild dementia cases in the community (Pond et al., 2018).

ASSESSMENT

No single diagnostic test can determine if a person has an NCD, and there are no widely accepted evidence-based guidelines for assessment of NCDs; therefore, a careful history and physical examination, laboratory testing, and imaging should be used to guide the clinical examination. Throughout the evaluation, it is important to consider possibilities for reversible causes of behavior changes.

The history should include subjective data from reports and patient-rated screening tools to obtain the patient's evaluations of their own cognitive capacity. The subjective information should be followed with objective data findings, including (a) neuropsychological testing; (b) observation of cognitive abilities (impairments in memory, language, orientation, recognition, and executive functions); and (c) an assessment of neuropsychiatric symptoms, such as apathy, agitation, psychosis (delusions and hallucinations), depression, anxiety, aggression, disinhibition, sleep disturbances, appetite changes, motor activity (fidgeting and pacing), repetitive vocalizations, wandering, restlessness, and refusal of care. Other resources include information from family members and other collateral sources and assessments from specialists, such as neurologists, neuropsychologists, geriatricians, and geriatric psychiatrists, all of whom use a variety of approaches and tools to help make a diagnosis. Additionally, the following laboratory tests can be used as a tool for diagnosis:

- B_{12} deficiency/serum vitamin B_{12} and folate level
- C-reactive protein
- Calcium level
- Complete blood count
- Complete metabolic panel
- Erythrocyte sedimentation rate
- Folate deficiency
- Glucose
- HIV
- Liver function test
- Neurosyphilis
- Thyroid-stimulating hormone
- Toxicology screening (urine/serum)

DIAGNOSTIC WORKUP

The diagnostic workup for NCDs typically begins in primary-care settings. Early and accurate diagnosis of NCDs enables patients and families to access supportive interventions and plan future care needs. Furthermore, early diagnosis promotes better patient outcomes. Before making a diagnosis, practitioners should assess the patient's diet, nutrition, and use of alcohol and conduct a neurologic exam to test reflexes, coordination, muscle tone and strength, eye movement, speech, and sensation.

BRIEF COGNITIVE SCREENING USING VALIDATED TOOLS

The diagnosis of NCD dementia cannot be solely based on a low score on a brief screening assessment; however, these screenings help to quantify the types and severity of impairment. Clinicians in primary-care settings use brief cognitive screenings to detect memory dysfunction. These evaluations should be guided by the scope of the patient's, family members', or clinician's concerns. Initial testing for cognitive concerns requires a mental status examination (MSE); cognitive and behavioral assessments using screening tools such as the MMSE, Mini-Cog, and

Montreal Cognitive Assessment (MoCA); and, if warranted, formal neuropsychological testing.

Essential Facts

Factors influencing decline for individuals with dementia include the following:

- Medical comorbidities
- Sedation
- Limited engagement in physical activity and meaningful interactions

THE MENTAL STATUS EXAMINATION

The MSE is a systematic and structured assessment that reports the following:

- The clinician's reaction to the patient
- The patient's appearance and general behavior
- The patient's attitude and insight
- The patient's cognitive abilities, including attention, language memory, constructional ability, and abstract reasoning
- The patient's level of consciousness and attentiveness/state of wakefulness
- The patient's mood and affect
- The patient's motor and speech activity
- The patient's thoughts and perceptions

MINI-MENTAL STATE EXAMINATION

The MMSE is a quick and simple test with high psychometrical properties, especially reliability. The MMSE includes a series of questions to test a range of skills and to detect cognitive deficits in attention, memory, and language functions. The maximum MMSE score is 30 points, and a score of 20 to 24 suggests mild dementia. A MMSE score of 13 to 20 suggests moderate dementia, and a score of less than 12 indicates severe dementia.

MINI-COG

The Mini-Cog, an initial screening test for dementia, is a brief assessment that takes approximately 3 to 5 minutes to complete. The test consists of a memory task that involves recall of three words or common objects and an evaluation of a clock-drawing task.

MONTREAL COGNITIVE ASSESSMENT

The MoCA tests subtle cognitive deficits typical in the early stages of dementia. The MoCA also requires patients to complete complex tasks to assess short-term memory; visuospatial abilities; executive functions; attention, concentration, and working memory; language; and orientation to time and place.

ADDITIONAL ADULT AND OLDER ADULT SCREENING TOOLS

According to Cordell et al. (2013), there is no single cognition assessment tool considered to be the gold standard in diagnosing dementia. However, the following valid and reliable tools are referenced in the literature:

- Caregiver Assessment Tools
- Eight-Item Informant Interview to Differentiate Aging and Dementia
- General Practitioner Assessment of Cognition
- Memory Impairment Screen
- Mini-Cog
- Short Form of the Informant Questionnaire on Cognitive Decline in the Elderly
- Short Informant Questionnaire on Cognitive Decline in the Elderly

STRUCTURAL BRAIN IMAGING

Evidence has shown that CT or MRI should be used to exclude other cerebral pathologies, such as tumors, strokes, damage from trauma, fluid, and vascular and frontotemporal degenerative etiologies. CT and MRI can also help identify treatable causes, such as subdural hematoma and normal pressure hydrocephalus (O'Brien et al., 2017). Brain imaging can be especially useful in cases where dementia is of recent onset and is rapidly progressing; younger onset dementia (65 years of age); history of head trauma; or neurologic symptoms suggesting focal disease (Cordell et al., 2013; O'Brien et al., 2017). Although not diagnostic for AD, neuroimaging has shown to be supportive in the evaluation of NCDs. Information from MRIs, CT scans, and PET brain scans for beta-amyloid protein can be used to support biomarkers and cerebrospinal fluid levels of amyloid and phosphorylated tau. Table 10.5 provides a risk assessment for clinicians to use for patients with neurocognitive conditions.

Essential Facts

Clinicians should conduct a cerebrospinal fluid examination if Creutzfeldt–Jakob disease or rapidly progressive dementia is suspected.

Essential Facts

Neuropsychiatric symptoms such as delusions, hallucinations, agitation, anxiety, apathy, disinhibition, irritability, and aberrant motor behavior may worsen as NCDs progress.

Table 10.5

Patient Assessment for Neurocognitive Conditions

Area of Assessment	Considerations
Environment	■ Noise ■ New caregiver
Behavior and cognitive changes	■ Medications (prescription and over the counter) ■ Infections ■ Toxic metabolic causes of delirium ■ Pain ■ Constipation ■ Urinary retention ■ Visual and auditory impairment
Mood assessment	■ Assess for depression or other mood disorders ■ Assess for memory problems, loss of interest in life, and other symptoms that overlap
Risk of harm	■ Carefully assess risk of harm to self and others ■ Assess and note the type, frequency, severity, pattern, and timing of symptoms

FURTHER ASSESSMENT

The list that follows contains is useful clinical data in the safety risk assessment of individuals with dementia or other neurocognitive conditions:

- Activities of daily living (ADLs)
- Housing
- Level of education
- Personal care
- Psychiatric and medical history (including recent surgeries)
- Psychologic measures
- Substance and medication use

Atypical Presentation (Patients Younger Than 60 Years; Rapidly Progressive Dementia)

Additional testing may be required in patients who present atypical presentations of sudden onset of cognitive changes.

- Electroencephalography
- Lumbar puncture
- May benefit from a more extensive evaluation
- Serologic tests

DIAGNOSTIC CHALLENGES

Neurocognitive impairments that present without distinctive neurologic signs or evidence of medical or neurologic disease can create diagnostic challenges, such as the following:

- Delays in diagnostic evaluation
- Early stages of dementia remain underdetected or underdiagnosed
- Gaps in knowledge, skills, confidence, attitudes, and resources among caregivers and clinicians
- Lack of diagnostic resources
- Patient often has little insight and does not notice symptoms
- Stigma around AD or reluctance to report signs or symptoms
- Time burden associated with testing and counseling

Essential Facts

Psychosocial interventions that are person centered, individually tailored, and noninvasive may be more effective at improving mood, reducing agitation, and addressing depression and anxiety for people with dementia (Annear et al., 2015).

Essential Facts

According to Cordell et al. (2013), 81% of individuals who meet the criteria for dementia have never received a documented diagnosis.

MEDICATION PRESCRIBING CONSIDERATIONS

The U.S. Food and Drug Administration (FDA) has approved medications to treat symptoms of dementia caused by AD. These drugs provide short-term relief from cognitive dementia symptoms, and some can also help slow the progression of AD-related dementia. According to Annear et al. (2015), the potential for harm in the use of medication should be weighed carefully against the impact on quality of life for people diagnosed with dementia. Due to the nature of NCDs, older adults with cognitive deficits who are prescribed medications are at an increased risk for medication-taking errors and nonadherence that can lead to negative health outcomes. Additionally, due to comorbid illness, polypharmacy risks must be assessed. Tables 10.6 through 10.8 provide FDA-approved medications in the management of neurocognitive conditions, including acetylcholinesterase inhibitors (AChEI), N-Methyl-D-Aspartate (NMDA) antagonists, and amyloid beta-directed antibody treatment.

Cognitive Enhancer Drugs

According to the cholinergic hypothesis, the chief cause of AD is the reduction in acetylcholine (ACh) synthesis; therefore, acetylcholinesterase (AChE) is a treatment strategy to increase the cholinergic levels in the brain by inhibiting or delaying the breakdown of ACh released into synaptic clefts and increasing cholinergic neurotransmission to improve the symptoms of dementia (Birks et al., 2015). Because ACh is also found in other areas of the body, these drugs

Table 10.6

Acetylcholinesterase Inhibitors

Generic Name (Brand Name)	Dosage Forms	FDA Approval	Clinical Considerations
Donepezil (Aricept)	Tablets OD Tablets	*Adults:* Alzheimer's disease *Non-FDA Uses*: prophylaxis, multi-infarct dementia *Pediatrics:* safety in pediatric use has not been established. *Older Adult Considerations:* *,**	This is the first-line medication used.
Rivastigmine (Exelon)	Capsules Solution Topical Patch	*Adults:* dementia of Alzheimer's disease in mild, moderate, and severe cases (only patches indicated for severe cases), dementia of Parkinson's disease in mild and moderate cases *Non-FDA Uses*: prophylaxis, multi-infarct dementia *Pediatrics:* safety in pediatric use has not been established *Older Adult Considerations*: *,**	Oral should be taken with meals.
Galantamine (Razadyne, Razadyne ER, Reminyl)	Tablets Solution ER Capsules	*Adults:* dementia of Alzheimer's disease in mild, moderate, and severe cases *Non-FDA Uses*: cerebrovascular disease (Alzheimer's disease), multi-infarct dementia *Pediatrics:* safety in pediatric use has not been established *Older Adult Considerations*: *,**	Monitor renal and hepatic function.

*Follow standard adult dosing.
**Associated with syncope, bradycardia, increased fall risk.
ER, extended release; FDA, U.S. Food and Drug Administration; OD, orally disintegrating

Table 10.7

Types of N-Methyl-D-Aspartate Antagonists

Generic Name (Brand Name)	Type	Dosage Forms	FDA Approval	Clinical Considerations
Memantine (Namenda, Namenda XR)	N-Methyl-D-Aspartate (NMDA) Antagonist	Tablets Solution XR Capsule	*Adults:* dementia of Alzheimer's disease in moderate to severe cases *Pediatrics:* safety in pediatric use has not been established *Older Adult Considerations:* *	Monitor hepatic function. Medical conditions that increase urine pH levels can increase drug plasma levels due to decreased urinary elimination.
Memantine/ Donepezil (Namzaric ER)	Combination AcetylcholinesTerase Inhibitors (AChEI)/N-Methyl-D-Aspartate Antagonists	Donepezil/ Memantine Capsule	*Adults:* moderate to severe Alzheimer's disease *Non-FDA Uses:* mild to moderate Alzheimer's disease *Pediatrics:* safety in pediatric use has not been established	Take in the evening

*Follow standard adult dosing. Associated with syncope, bradycardia, increased fall risk.
FDA, U.S. Food and Drug Administration.

Table 10.8

Amyloid Beta-Directed Antibody

Generic Name (Brand Name)	Dosage Forms	FDA Approval	Clinical Considerations
Aducanumab (Aduhlem)	Injectable Solution	*Adults:* Alzheimer's disease, mild cognitive impairment, or mild dementia stage of disease *Pediatrics:* safety in pediatric use has not been established	Refer to medication insert for monitoring guidelines —recent (within 1 year) brain MRI prior to initiating treatment and prior to seventh treatment.

FDA, U.S. Food and Drug Administration.

may cause unwanted effects. Additionally, donepezil inhibits both AchE activity and Aβ aggregation, a proteolytic fragment originated from amyloid precursor protein factors involved in AD pathogenesis (Sharma, 2019).

There are two main types of treatment: ChEI drugs and memantine, a glutamate receptor antagonist. According to O'Brien et al. (2017), combination therapy using a ChEI initially with the later addition of memantine is considered an optimal treatment for dementia as it advances (Sharma, 2019).

Memantine is prescribed to improve thinking, increase ability to carry on normal daily activities, and the decrease severity of behavior and mood problems among people with memory disorders (McShane et al., 2019). Aggressive behaviors, agitation, anxiety, and psychosis are symptoms that affect many people with NCDs. These symptoms are most commonly treated with antipsychotic drugs (see Chapter 7). Antipsychotic drug therapy should be a short-term treatment option only for those with severe symptoms.

BEHAVIORAL AND EDUCATIONAL INTERVENTIONS TO HELP WITH MEDICATION COMPLIANCE

The list that follows provides educational and behavioral interventions to improve medication adherence in individuals with dementia:

- Adherence monitoring with or without feedback
- Alarm/beeper
- Calendar/diary
- Contracting (verbal or written agreement)
- Follow-up (home visit, scheduled clinic visit, video/teleconferencing)
- Large print labels
- Multicompartment pillbox
- Reminder chart/medication list
- Reminders (mail, telephone, email)
- Simplification of medication regimens
- Skill-building programs

TARGET TREATMENT GOALS

According to Annear et al. (2015), there is no cure for dementia; therefore, management options should be measured against the impact on the quality of life, and nonpharmacologic interventions can be used to improve quality of life and ameliorate behavioral and psychologic symptoms of dementia. Treatment goals must address medical care and overall health, such as emotional well-being, maintaining independence, addressing needed services, and caregiver support. Dementia is a progressive condition that affects people across multiple domains; therefore, advanced care planning is required to address individual goals from the onset of diagnosis, and these goals must be continuously monitored and reviewed with the patient, caregivers, and treatment team. Person-centered care and the maintenance of close relationships during the early and later stages of dementia are required to recognize and address behavioral changes, memory impairments, and difficulties with executive functioning.

AIMS AND TREATMENT GOALS

Aims and goals for those suffering from dementia include the following:

- Aging and dying with dignity
- Assessments of coexisting or treatable physical and psychiatric symptoms (depression, pain, delirium)
- Lowering caregiver strain
- Managing behavioral symptoms
- Meaningful activity
- Ongoing assessments for comorbid conditions and changes in personal events
- Planning future care needs based on individual preferences
- Prevention of elder abuse (not being taken advantage of by others)
- Safety education (e.g., avoid falls, household hazards, or getting lost)
- Social interaction
- Supporting functional independence

BEHAVIORIAL THERAPY

Psychoeducation and psychotherapy such as cognitive behavioral therapy, an evidence-based psychosocial intervention designed to change dysfunctional thoughts and behavior, can be used to reduce symptom severity for individuals with comorbid anxiety and depression. Therapy that includes cognitive stimulation activities, such as puzzles, word games, indoor gardening, discussions of the past/reminiscence therapy, and cooking, has been shown to be beneficial. Moreover, occupational therapists can evaluate home environments and help patients and their caregivers develop compensatory strategies for ADLs to meet the patient's abilities. Occupational therapists can also develop environmental strategies to help adapt the patient's environment to their cognitive limitations.

MAINTENANCE PHASE OF TREATMENT

Ongoing assessments are needed to assess cognitive performance or ability to maintain ADLs. Clinicians should inquire about problems related to home activities, hobbies, and personal care.

Essential Facts

The Institute of Medicine (IOM) recommends that interprofessional teams be structured to maximize the skills and abilities of every team member and include clear goals with measurable outcomes for individuals with complex needs (Galvin et al., 2014).

DOMAINS FOR ONGOING MONITORING

Neurocognitive conditions are complex brain syndromes with a large spectrum of cognitive, functional, behavioral, and psychologic symptoms that require ongoing clinical monitoring for both patients and caregivers. The following should be monitored:

- ADLs
- Behavioral disturbance and mood changes (anxiety, depression, agitation)
- Caregiver burden
- Cognitive function (as measured by psychometric tests)
- Death and dying (values, beliefs, dignity)
- Dependency (such as institutionalization)
- Direct and indirect costs of management
- Effect on career
- Exercise and physical activity
- Quality of life
- Safety as measured by the overall incidence of adverse effects

CRITERIA FOR REFERRAL

Early diagnosis of dementia is crucial because treatments are more effective in the early stages of dementia. Earlier diagnosis and timely interventions provide health, financial, and social benefits for individuals and their caregivers. Referrals are warranted when the onset of dementia is within the preceding 6 months and the dementia is rapidly progressing. Additionally, clinicians can make referrals for social support services and specialist treatments to help individuals and caregivers understand and cope with the challenging symptoms of dementia. Notable side effects of dementia include the following:

- Elder abuse
- Extreme mood or personality changes
- Functional decline
- Increasing agitation or extremely bothered by hallucinations
- Medication side effects
- Psychosis
- Risk of suicide or hurting themselves or others
- Symptom control has not been attainable as outpatient

SUMMARY

NCDs have a high economic impact and place significant burdens on patients, caregivers, providers, and healthcare delivery systems; therefore, a comprehensive approach to dementia diagnosis is required to promote optimal outcomes. Additionally, the pharmacologic management of dementia is limited; thus, an evaluation of alternative approaches to healthcare delivery is warranted. Team-based, collaborative care models provide pragmatic strategies to best meet the needs of patients and families.

RESOURCES

- Alzheimer's Disease International: www.alzint.org/what-we-do/policy/dementia-plans
- World Health Organization (WHO): Guidelines on risk reduction of cognitive decline and dementia https://www.who.int/publications/i/item/9789241550543
- World Health Organization (WHO): A guide toward a dementia plan https://www.who.int/publications/i/item/9789241514132
- World Health Organization (WHO): The global dementia observatory reference guide https://apps.who.int/iris/handle/10665/272669
- U.S. Preventive Services Task Force (USPSTF): Final recommendation statement on cognitive impairment in older adults—Screening https://www.uspreventiveservicestaskforce.org/uspstf/document/RecommendationStatementFinal/cognitive-impairment-in-older-adults-screening
- American Academy of Neurology (AAN): Practice parameter: Evaluation and management of driving risk in dementia, update https://www.ncbi.nlm.nih.gov/pmc/articles/PMC2860481/
- American College of Radiology (ACR): ACR Appropriateness Criteria on dementia https://acsearch.acr.org/docs/3111292/Narrative/
- American Academy of Neurology (AAN): Practice guideline on mild cognitive impairment, update https://www.aan.com/Guidelines/Home/GetGuidelineContent/882
- American Psychiatric Association (APA): Practice guideline on the use of antipsychotics to treat agitation or psychosis in patients with dementia https://psychiatryonline.org/doi/pdf/10.1176/appi.books.9780890426807
- American College of Radiology (ACR)—American Society of Neuroradiology (ASNR): Practice parameter for brain PET/CT imaging in dementia https://www.acr.org/-/media/ACR/Files/Practice-Parameters/brain-pet-ct-dementia.pdf
- American Geriatrics Society (AGS): Feeding tubes in advanced dementia position statement https://agsjournals.onlinelibrary.wiley.com/doi/10.1111/jgs.12924
- National Institute on Aging (NIA)—Alzheimer's Association (ALZ): Guidelines for the neuropathologic assessment of Alzheimer's disease—A practical approach
- American Psychological Association (APA): Guidelines for the evaluation of dementia and age-related cognitive change https://www.apa.org/practice/guidelines/guidelines-dementia-age-related-cognitive-change.pdf

REVIEW QUESTIONS

1. According to the cholinergic hypothesis, a primary cause for Alzheimer's disease (AD) is which one of the following?
   a. Changes in acetylcholine synthesis
   b. Increased synaptic activity

c. Norepinephrine breakdown in the synaptic cleft
d. Delay in the breakdown of dopamine in the synaptic cleft

2. Which one of the statements below is false?
   a. There is no cure for dementia.
   b. Treatments are more effective in the early stages of dementia.
   c. Memantine is an acetylcholinesterase inhibitor.
   d. Antipsychotics can help with agitation and psychosis in older adults with dementia.
3. Behavioral and educational interventions to help with medication compliance can include which one of the following?
   a. Reminders (mail, telephone, email), multicompartment pillboxes, and large-print labels
   b. Simplification of medication regimens and contracting (verbal or written agreement)
   c. Alarm/beeper, skill-building programs, adherence monitoring
   d. All of the above help with medication compliance
4. Which one of the following statements is false?
   a. Individuals with Alzheimer's disease (AD) with the apolipoprotein E (APOE4) isoform have accelerated onset of dementia, worsened memory functioning, and higher amyloid β plaque burden than those who are not APOE4 carriers.
   b. Vascular dementia is the second most common form of dementia after Alzheimer's disease. It's caused when decreased blood flow damages brain tissue.
   c. Individuals with Lewy body dementia typically have onset of dementia symptoms and parkinsonian symptoms that appear closer together compared to those with Parkinson's dementia.
   d. All of the above statements are true.
5. Risk factors for dementia include which one of the following?
   a. Lower education attainment, hearing impairment, and lower cholesterol levels
   b. Increased air pollution and having a first-degree relative with Alzheimer's disease (AD)
   c. *APOE4* gene possession and being male
   d. All of the following are increased risk factors

REFERENCES

American Psychiatric Association. (2013). *Diagnostic and statistical manual of mental disorders* (5th ed.). https://doi.org/10.1176/appi.books.9780890425596

Annear, M. J., Toye, C., McInerney, F., Eccleston, C., Tranter, B., Elliott, K. E., & Robinson, A. (2015). What should we know about dementia in the 21st century? A Delphi consensus study. *BMC Geriatrics*, *15*, Article 5. https://doi.org/10.1186/s12877-015-0008-1

Birks, J. S., Chong, L. Y., & Grimley Evans, J. (2015). Rivastigmine for Alzheimer's disease. *The Cochrane Database of Systematic Reviews*, *9*(9), Article CD001191. https://doi.org/10.1002/14651858.CD001191.pub4

Chakrabarty, T., Hadjipavlou, G., & Lam, R. W. (2016). Cognitive dysfunction in major depressive disorder: Assessment, impact, and management. *Focus*, *14*(2), 194–206. https://doi.org/10.1176/appi.focus.20150043

Cordell, C. B., Borson, S., Boustani, M., Chodosh, J., Reuben, D., Verghese, J., Thies, W., Fried, L. B., & Medicare Detection of Cognitive Impairment Workgroup. (2013). Alzheimer's Association recommendations for operationalizing the detection of cognitive impairment during the Medicare Annual Wellness Visit in a primary care setting. *Alzheimer's & Dementia*, *9*(2), 141–150. https://doi.org/10.1016/j.jalz.2012.09.011

Galvin, J. E., Valois, L., & Zweig, Y. (2014). Collaborative transdisciplinary team approach for dementia care. *Neurodegenerative Disease Management*, *4*(6), 455–469. https://doi.org/10.2217/nmt.14.47

GBD 2016 Dementia Collaborators. (2019). Global, regional, and national burden of Alzheimer's disease and other dementias, 1990–2016: A systematic analysis for the Global Burden of Disease Study 2016. *The Lancet Neurology*, *18*(1), 88–106. https://doi.org/10.1016/S1474-4422(18)30403-4

Henderson, M. X., Trojanowski, J. Q., & Lee, V. M. (2019). α-Synuclein pathology in Parkinson's disease and related α-synucleinopathies. *Neuroscience Letters*, *709*, Article 134316. https://doi.org/10.1016/j.neulet.2019.134316

James, B. D., & Bennett, D. A. (2019). Causes and patterns of dementia: An update in the era of redefining Alzheimer's disease. *Annual Review of Public Health*, *40*, 65–84. https://doi.org/10.1146/annurev-publhealth-040218-043758

Livingston, G., Huntley, J., Sommerlad, A., Ames, D., Ballard, C., Banerjee, S., Brayne, C., Burns, A., Cohen-Mansfield, J., Cooper, C., Costafreda, S. G., Dias, A., Fox, N., Gitlin, L. N., Howard, R., Kales, H. C., Kivimäki, M., Larson, E. B., Ogunniyi, A., … Mukadam, N. (2020). Dementia prevention, intervention, and care: 2020 report of the Lancet Commission. *The Lancet Commissions*, *396*(10248), 413–446. https://doi.org/10.1016/S0140-6736(20)30367-6

McShane, R., Westby, M. J., Roberts, E., Minakaran, N., Schneider, L., Farrimond, L. E., Maayan, N., Ware, J., & Debarros, J. (2019). Memantine for dementia. *The Cochrane Database of Systematic Reviews*, *3*(3), Article CD003154. https://doi.org/10.1002/14651858.CD003154.pub6

O'Brien, J. T., Holmes, C., Jones, M., Jones, R., Livingston, G., McKeith, I., Mittler, P., Passmore, P., Ritchie, C., Robinson, L., Sampson, E. L., Taylor, J. P., Thomas, A., & Burns, A. (2017). Clinical practice with anti-dementia drugs: A revised (third) consensus statement from the British Association for Psychopharmacology. *Journal of Psychopharmacology*, *31*(2), 147–168. https://doi.org/10.1177/0269881116680924

Piers, R., Albers, G., Gilissen, J., De Lepeleire, J., Steyaert, J., Van Mechelen, W., Steeman, E., Dillen, L., Vanden Berghe, P., & Van den Block, L. (2018). Advance care planning in dementia: Recommendations for healthcare professionals. *BMC Palliative Care*, *17*(1), Article 88. https://doi.org/10.1186/s12904-018-0332-2

Pond, D., Mate, K., Stocks, N., Gunn, J., Disler, P., Magin, P., Marley, J., Paterson, N., Horton, G., Goode, S., Weaver, N., & Brodaty, H. (2018). Effectiveness of a peer-mediated educational intervention in improving general practitioner diagnostic assessment and management of dementia: A cluster randomised controlled trial. *BMJ Open*, *8*(8), Article e021125. https://doi.org/10.1136/bmjopen-2017-021125

Raulin, A. C., Kraft, L., Al-Hilaly, Y. K., Xue, W. F., McGeehan, J. E., Atack, J. R., & Serpell, L. (2019). The molecular basis for apolipoprotein E4 as the major risk factor for late-onset Alzheimer's disease. *Journal of Molecular Biology*, *431*(12), 2248–2265. https://doi.org/10.1016/j.jmb.2019.04.019

Sachdev, P. S., Mohan, A., Taylor, L., & Jeste, D. V. (2015). *DSM-5* and mental disorders in older individuals: An overview. *Harvard Review of Psychiatry*, *23*(5), 320–328. https://doi.org/10.1097/HRP.0000000000000090

Sharma, K. (2019). Cholinesterase inhibitors as Alzheimer's therapeutics (review). *Molecular Medicine Reports*, *20*(2), 1479–1487. https://doi.org/10.3892/mmr.2019.10374

Williams, T., Borchelt, D. R., & Chakrabarty, P. (2020). Therapeutic approaches targeting Apolipoprotein E function in Alzheimer's disease. *Molecular Neurodegeneration*, *15*(1), Article 8. https://doi.org/10.1186/s13024-020-0358-9

11

Sleep Disorders

Sleep is an innate biologic requirement for human life that plays a key role in mental and physical health. Restful sleep reverses oxidative stress, repletes energy stores, is vital to learning and memory, and impacts overall functioning. In the United States, approximately 30% of adults report that they sleep less than 7 hours per 24 hours and are chronically sleep deprived. Additionally, approximately 50% to 80% of adults with mental illnesses report difficulties with falling or staying asleep (Seow et al., 2018; Slavish et al., 2019). Sleep disturbance and mental health conditions are closely intertwined; disrupted sleep is either a symptom or a consequence of a mental health condition (Freeman et al., 2017), and disturbed sleep is a contributory factor in the occurrence of mental health disorders (Mead & Irish, 2020). This chapter provides a brief overview of insomnia along with the causes of, evidence in assessing, and how to diagnose, treat, and manage insomnia.

In this chapter you will learn:

1. How to determine the specific manifestations of sleep disorders
2. How to compare pharmacologic options for insomnia and sleep-related disorders
3. How to name five key features of insomnia and related disorders
4. How to identify screening tools for sleep disorders
5. How to consider medication safety in prescribing for and managing insomnia and related disorders
6. How to assess therapeutic responses in sleep and related disorders

SLEEP OVERVIEW

Difficulties with either sleep initiation or sleep maintenance have been linked to emotional, behavioral, genetic, and environmental influences and biologic or circadian disruption factors. Poor sleep has been associated with increased rates of morbidity and mortality (Mead & Irish, 2020) because insufficient sleep or poor sleep quality can negatively impact general health, cardiovascular health, metabolic health, mental health, immunologic health, human performance, cancer, pain, hormone regulation, gene expression, and mortality (Slavish et al., 2019; Watson et al., 2015; Worley, 2018). Individual factors that influence a person's sleep include genetics, knowledge, attitudes, environment, socioeconomic status, employment, religion, ethnicity, and beliefs about the relationship between sleep and one's overall health. Despite the public health consequences of insufficient sleep, insomnia, and other associated sleep conditions, there is still a lot to be learned about the intricacies of how sleep works. Sleep health continues to be underrecognized by practicing clinicians, and a lack of consensus exists for pharmacologic nonmanagement approaches to sleep-related conditions.

The National Institute of Mental Health stated that "sleep and wakefulness are endogenous, recurring, behavioral states that reflect coordinated changes in the dynamic functional organization of the brain and that optimize physiology, behavior, and health. Homeostatic and circadian processes regulate the propensity for wakefulness and sleep" (as cited in Buysse, 2014, p. 10). In other words, sleep–wake homeostasis, the circadian alerting system, and environmental factors regulate the body's need for sleep and wakefulness. During sleep states, the brain cycles through different stages that are the basis for sleep evaluation and diagnosis. Stages of sleep are referred to as nonrapid eye movement (NREM) sleep and rapid eye movement (REM) sleep. NREM sleep is also referred to as quiet sleep, whereas REM sleep, the stage where dreaming occurs, is referred to as active sleep (Huang et al., 2021).

Wakefulness is characterized as a behavioral state during which an individual exhibits voluntary motor activation and is responsive to internal and external stimuli (Buysse, 2014). The International Classification of Sleep Disorders classifications include (a) disorders of initiating and maintaining sleep (insomnias), (b) disorders of excessive somnolence, (c) disorders of sleep–wake schedule, and (d) dysfunctions associated with sleep, sleep stages, partial arousal, or parasomnias (Cormier, 1990). The *Diagnostic and Statistical Manual of Mental Disorders* (5th ed.; *DSM-5*; American Psychiatric Association [APA], 2013) recognizes 12 sleep–wake disorders based on the International Classification of Sleep Disorders by taking into consideration the pathological and etiologic factors associated with sleep–wake conditions (Seow et al., 2018).

Approximately 30% of adults in the United States report difficulty initiating or maintaining sleep, waking up too early, or experiencing nonrestorative sleep (Slavish et al., 2019). According to Freeman et al. (2017), the most common form of sleep disorder is insomnia, which is characterized as ongoing difficulties in initiating and/or staying asleep that result in excessive daytime sleepiness and is strongly associated with psychiatric conditions, with more than 90% of individuals with major depressive disorder (MDD) having an insomnia-related sleep disturbance (Seow et al., 2018). Daytime symptoms of insomnia include the following:

- Behavioral problems, hyperactivity, and impulsivity
- Concerns or dissatisfaction with sleep
- Daytime sleepiness
- Fatigue, malaise, and low energy
- Headaches
- Impaired social, family, vocational, or academic performance
- Increased errors or accidents
- Low attention, poor concentration, or memory impairment
- Mood disturbance or irritability
- Physical deconditioning
- Reduced motivation, energy, and initiative
- Sexual dysfunction
- Weight gain or loss

Essential Facts

- There is a bidirectional relationship between insomnia and psychiatric disorders.
- According to Seow et al. (2018), MDD, bipolar disorder (BD), and anxiety disorders such as posttraumatic stress disorder (PTSD) and schizophrenia spectrum disorder are strongly associated with insomnia.

Essential Facts

Sleep–Wake Homeostasis and the Circadian System Regulation

The following parts of the brain are involved in sleep–wake homeostasis and the circadian system:

- Amygdala
- Basal forebrain
- Cerebral cortex
- Hypothalamus
- Midbrain
- Pineal gland
- Thalamus
- Brainstem

Neuromodulators involved in sleep–wake homeostasis and the circadian system are as follows:

- Acetylcholine
- Adenosine
- Gamma aminobutyric acid (GABA)
- Orexin
- Serotonin

(*continued*)

Essential Facts (*continued*)

Sleep-related hormones are as follows:

- Adrenaline
- Cortisol
- Ghrelin
- Growth hormone
- Leptin
- Melatonin
- Norepinephrine

Essential Facts

Infants require approximately twice the amount of sleep time as mature adults.

Essential Facts

Wakefulness can be characterized as a behavioral state during which an individual exhibits voluntary motor activation and is responsive to internal and external stimuli.

Essential Facts

Obstructive sleep apnea is the most common breathing-related sleep disorder (Rezaie et al., 2021). According to Kapur et al. (2017), polysomnography is the standard diagnostic test for the diagnosis of obstructive sleep apnea in adults.

DIAGNOSTIC CRITERIA

Given their ubiquity in clinical practice settings, the *DSM-5* sleep–wake disorders classification measures aim to assist practitioners in identifying and facilitating the differential diagnosis of sleep–wake complaints and clarify when a referral to a sleep disorders specialist is warranted. The core features of each sleep-related disorder relate to the patient's dissatisfaction regarding the quality, timing, and amount of sleep accompanied with daytime distress and functional impairment. Table 11.1 provides the diagnostic criteria and key features of sleep–wake disorders.

Table 11.1

Diagnostic Criteria and Key Features of Sleep–Wake Disorders Diagnostic Groups

Disorder	Features
Insomnia disorder	A disorder of hyperarousal or dissatisfaction with sleep duration or quality plus one or more of the following characteristics: ▪ Occurs in settings of adequate opportunity ▪ Difficulty falling asleep, remaining asleep, early morning awakening ▪ Causes distress or impairment in functioning >3 nights/week in >3 months ▪ Not better explained by another condition, substance, or coexisting condition ▪ Acute: persists 1 to 7 days ▪ Chronic: persists ≥ 1 month
Hypersomnolence disorder narcolepsy	Excessive sleepiness (hypersomnolence) despite having slept ≥7 hours, plus one or more of the following characteristics: ▪ Recurrent periods of sleep during the day ▪ Sleeping >9 hours and not feeling rested ▪ Difficulty being fully awake after sleeping ▪ Occurs at least 3 times per week for at least 3 months ▪ Causes distress or impairment in functioning ▪ Not better explained by another condition, substance, or coexisting condition
Breathing-related sleep disorders ▪ Obstructive sleep apnea ▪ Central sleep apnea ▪ Sleep-related hypoventilation ▪ Sleep-related hypoxemia disorder	▪ Abnormal respiration during sleep ▪ Partial or complete closure of the upper airway, resulting in disturbed breathing of airflow for ≥10 seconds during sleep ▪ Gold standard: polysomnographic assessment ▪ Associated with decreased quality of life and significant medical comorbidities
Circadian rhythm sleep–wake disorders ▪ Delayed sleep phase type ▪ Advanced sleep phase type ▪ Irregular sleep–wake type ▪ Non-24-hour sleep–wake type ▪ Shift-work type ▪ Unspecified type	▪ Sleep and wakefulness occurring at abnormal or irregular times due to an alteration of one's circadian system ▪ Sleep disturbance leads to daytime sleepiness ▪ Causes distress or impairment in functioning ▪ Episodic: symptoms 1 to 3 months ▪ Persistent: symptoms ≥3 months ▪ Recurrent: ≥2 episodes within a year
Parasomnias ▪ NREM ▪ Sleep arousal disorders (sleepwalking type/sleep terror type) ▪ Nightmare disorder ▪ REM sleep behavior disorder ▪ Restless legs syndrome	▪ Recurrent episodes of unusual or odd behavioral, experiential, or physiologic events occurring during sleep, specific sleep stages, or sleep–wake transitions ▪ Not attributable to the physiologic effects of a substance ▪ Not better explained by coexisting mental and medical disorders

(*continued*)

Table 11.1

Diagnostic Criteria and Key Features of Sleep–Wake Disorders Diagnostic Groups (*continued*)

Disorder	Features
▪ Substance/medication-induced sleep disorder ▪ Other specified insomnia disorder ▪ Unspecified insomnia disorder ▪ Other specified hypersomnolence disorder ▪ Unspecified hypersomnolence disorder ▪ Other specified sleep–wake disorder ▪ Unspecified sleep–wake disorder	

Essential Facts

Insomnia is identified as chronic when it has persisted for at least 3 months at a frequency of at least 3 times per week. When the insomnia meets the symptom criteria but has persisted for less than 3 months, it is considered short-term insomnia (Sateia et al., 2017).

Essential Facts

Women of all ages report more sleep problems than men.

INSOMNIA EVALUATION

Insomnia is primarily diagnosed by clinical evaluation through a detailed comprehensive sleep, medical, family, substance, and psychiatric history.

- Compile a detailed history:
  - Compile a detailed history from the patient, bed partner, or family member; collect a sleep questionnaire to assess sleep patterns and habits, medical conditions, and medications that influence sleep quality/quantity and level of daytime sleepiness.
- Investigate details about the chief complaint:
  - Start of symptoms; pattern since onset and associated factors including medical, environmental, occupational, psychologic/stress, and lifestyle choices; course of insomnia, including past help-seeking experience or insomnia-related sleep problems; previous diagnosis of any specific sleep disorder(s)

- Type of interventions and effectiveness of intervention (medications, counseling/therapies)
- Impact of the sleep complaint on the patient's life
- Type of symptoms to include restless legs sensation (periodic limb or excessive movements during sleep); snoring, or witnessed apneic episodes; night sweating, coughing, gasping/choking/snorting, dryness of the mouth, or bruxism; any abnormal behaviors during sleep; daytime sleepiness; presence of cataplexy; sleep paralysis; and hypnagogic or hypnapompic hallucinations

- Inquire about meal and sleep schedules, caffeine intake, alcohol, and nicotine use, as well as use of illicit drugs.
- Review pertinent medical/surgical/psychiatric history and past treatment efficacy or lack thereof.
- Determine if there is any family history of sleep disorders.
- Have patient complete a 2-week sleep log; this is a helpful method to track sleep information.
- Review the history of polysomnography results, the gold-standard measure of sleep.
- Determine if the insomnia is associated with comorbid mental or physical conditions.
- Determine if the insomnia is persistent or in isolation during certain time periods.
- Assess screen time prior to bed:
  - Sleep hygiene
  - Caffeine intake
  - Life events

An evaluation of an individual's sleep complaints may include the clinical interview, sleep diaries, questionnaires, actigraphy, polysomnography (laboratory or home), or other tests (see Table 11.2). Home-based technology monitoring enables patient and clinicians to accurately track the patient's treatment and modify therapy as needed.

Many questionnaires can be used to assess sleep. Questionnaires are used in clinical practice to provide subjective psychometric properties. Patient burden and clinical use often depend on instrument accessibility, appropriateness, and ease of administration.

PEDIATRIC AND ADOLESCENT SCREENING QUESTIONNAIRES

In primary-care outpatient settings, subjective sleep questionnaires are accessible and cost-effective assessments of sleep quality, daytime sleepiness, and sleep-related functional impairments.

INFANTS

Practitioners can use the Brief Infant Sleep Questionnaire to screen infants for sleep-related disorders.

Table 11.2

Laboratory Testing for Sleep Disorders: Key Features

Test	Features
Electroencephalogram	Measures sleep stages. Checks for abnormal brain activity, including seizures, during sleep.
Polysomnography: a study done while sleeping (laboratory or home based) that defines sleep and wake states and sleep stages based on standard criteria	May be used to rule out sleep disorders such as obstructive sleep apnea and for subtyping insomnia disorders. This is the gold-standard technique for sleep assessment.
Electrocardiogram	Monitors heart rate and checks for any abnormal heart rhythms.
Electromyography	Tracks REM sleep and measures muscle movement to assess for restless leg syndrome (unpleasant sensations in a person's legs and an irresistible urge to move them).
Actigraphy	Devices are worn on the wrist to record movements. Uses algorithms in computer software programs to estimate sleep parameters. Provides objective sleep information in the patient's natural sleep environment.
Breathing test	Assesses for respiratory problems, including issues with chest and abdominal movements and airflow through mouth and nose.
Multiple sleep latency test	Performed after a full-night polysomnography (after at least 6 hours of sleep) to measure the degree of daytime sleepiness to evaluate for possible narcolepsy.

REM, rapid eye movement

CHILDREN 1 YEAR OF AGE AND OLDER

Clinicians can use the following questionnaires to screen children aged 1 and older for sleep-related disorders:

- BEARS (B = Bedtime Issues, E = Excessive Daytime Sleepiness, A = Night Awakenings, R = Regularity and Duration of Sleep, S = Snoring)
- Children's Sleep Habits Questionnaire
- Cleveland Adolescent Sleepiness Questionnaire
- Epworth Sleepiness Scale, Revised for Children
- Habitual Activity Estimation Scale
- Pediatric Daytime Sleepiness Scale
- Pediatric Sleep Questionnaire
- Tayside Children's Sleep Questionnaire
- Ten-Item Sleep Screener

TO SCREEN ADULTS AND OLDER ADULTS FOR SLEEP ISSUES: SCREENING QUESTIONNAIRES

Clinicians can use the following questionnaires to screen children aged 1 and older for sleep issues:

- Calgary Sleep Apnea Quality of Life Index
- Cataplexy Questionnaire
- Insomnia Severity Index
- Pittsburgh Sleep Quality Index
- Restless Legs Syndrome Quality of Life Questionnaire
- Sleep Disorders Questionnaire
- The Berlin Questionnaire
- The Brief Insomnia Questionnaire
- The Epworth Sleepiness Scale
- The Flinders Fatigue Scale
- The Functional Outcomes of Sleep Questionnaire
- The Sleep Timing Questionnaire
- The STOP-BANG Questionnaire

The nonspecific nature of sleep-related symptoms, the limitations of diagnostic tests, and the high rates of comorbid conditions can make diagnosing sleep conditions difficult.

DIFFERENTIAL DIAGNOSIS

Treatment often focuses on the primary disorder; therefore, clinicians need to be cognizant that insomnia, characterized by regular sleep disturbances, an inability to fall asleep naturally, or persistent nightly waking, can be primary or secondary to another medical and/or psychologic condition. The list that follows contains commonly associated conditions associated with sleep–wake disorders.

- Insomnia due to a drug or substance
- Mood disorder
- Neurodevelopmental disorder
- Obstructive sleep apnea
- Periodic limb movement disorder
- Restless legs syndrome
- Sleeplessness and circadian rhythm disorder

Essential Facts

Standardized intake and screening questionnaires are used to assess sleep patterns and habits, medical conditions, medications that influence sleep quality/quantity, and level of daytime sleepiness.

DIAGNOSTIC CHALLENGES

The assessment and treatment of sleep conditions can be complex since poor or inadequate sleep can be associated with a multitude of conditions. Notably, reported sleep symptoms can be vague, characteristic which is of several sleep disorders, or be secondary to other medical or psychologic conditions. Additional clinical challenges in diagnosing sleep disturbances may include the amount of time required for thorough sleep assessments, difficulties in obtaining accurate information of sleep assessments, assessment bias, inaccuracy of patient reporting (i.e., by those with cognitive limitations, infants, and children; older patients and caregivers finding assessments to be cumbersome), lack of premorbid screening tools; and the multifactorial and complex causes for sleep symptoms.

Essential Facts

- No objective criteria exist for the diagnosis of insomnia disorder.
- Polysomnography is not indicated to diagnose insomnia disorder.

TARGET TREATMENT GOALS

The primary goal when addressing sleep issues is to provide efficient, sustainable, cost-effective, and patient-centered approaches to improve the health of patients, provide quality services, and improve clinical outcomes. Goals also include reduction of sleep and waking symptoms, improvement of daytime function, and the reduction of distress and impairments caused by the sleeping issue. It is important to educate patients on optimizing their sleep environment and to look for possible identifiable causes for the insomnia so that treatment can be focused on the root cause of the insomnia. For example, treat medical and psychiatric conditions with medications that do not interfere with sleep and take stimulating medications earlier in the day.

AN INTEGRATIVE APPROACH TO THE MANAGEMENT OF SLEEP ISSUES

Integrative therapies such as meditation, relaxation, yoga, massage, and music therapy are examples of supportive care for sleep-related disorder management.

- Acupuncture
- Art
- Environment
- Exercise
- Massage
- Mindfulness
- Music
- Nutrition
- Yoga
- Tai chi

MEDICATIONS FOR TREATMENT OF INSOMNIA IN PEDIATRIC AND ADULT POPULATIONS

The most widely used treatment for insomnia is pharmacologic therapy, including over-the-counter sleep aids and alcohol; however, no sleep-promoting medications have been clearly efficacious or indicated in the treatment of chronic insomnia (Sateia et al., 2017). When prescribing medications, continual management of comorbidities and nonpharmacologic interventions such as cognitive behavioral therapies for insomnia and sleep hygiene are considered first-line management options (Sateia et al., 2017). According to Sateia et al. (2017), pharmacotherapy should be considered within the context of specific treatment goals, comorbidities, prior treatment responses, availability, safety, patient preference, and cost considerations. Pharmacologic management options include benzodiazepines, nonbenzodiazepines, selective melatonin receptor agonists, selective histamine H-1 antagonists, the selective adrenergic α_1 antagonists, selective hypocretin/orexin antagonists, antidepressants, antipsychotics, and over-the-counter nonselective H-1 antagonists (Krystal, 2015). Tables 11.3 and 11.4 provide lists of U.S. Food and Drug Administration (FDA)-approved benzodiazepines and nonbenzodiazepines and dosages for insomnia treatment.

Essential Facts

Consider the following factors when prescribing a medication:

- High quality of evidence for efficacy
- Highly confident that benefits clearly outweigh harms
- Evidence that the effects of treatment are substantial without inflicting harm or too much risk to the patient

PRESCRIBING CONSIDERATIONS

After adequate assessment of cause and characteristics of sleep complaints, as well as evaluation and treatment of contributing comorbidities, treatment should be personalized depending on the type of sleep disturbance and the specific nature of each patient's insomnia. A risk–benefit ratio assessment is required when providing treatment, according to the traditional model of insomnia therapy. Clinicians need to assess the nonsleep adverse effects of medication administration, such as orthostatic hypotension and dizziness, fall precautions, and mental status (Krystal, 2015). Patients who are prescribed hypnotics should be counseled on the risks and management of drowsy driving.

Essential Facts

When considering sleep medications in older adults, the use of the American Geriatric Society Beers Criteria should be a starting point for improving medication appropriateness and safety.

Table 11.3

FDA-Approved Benzodiazepines Dosage for Insomnia

Generic Name (Brand Name)	Dosage Forms	FDA Approval	Clinical Considerations
Estazolam (ProSom)	Tablets	*Adults:* insomnia *Pediatrics:* safety in pediatric use has not been established *Older Adult Considerations:* ***	Take before bedtime.
Flurazepam (Dalmane)	Capsules	*Adults:* insomnia *Pediatrics:* insomnia (15 years and older) *Older Adult Considerations:* **,***	Take before bedtime.
Temazepam (Restoril)	Capsules	*Adults:* insomnia *Pediatrics:* safety in pediatric use has not been established *Older Adult Considerations:* **preferred benzodiazepine for older adults due to lack of active metabolite ***	Take before bedtime. Drug should be gradually tapered during discontinuation.
Triazolam (Halcion)	Tablet	*Adults:* insomnia *Pediatrics:* safety in pediatric use has not been established *Older Adult Considerations:* **,***	Take before bedtime.
Quazepam (Doral)	Tablet	*Adults:* insomnia *Pediatrics:* safety in pediatric use has not been established *Older Adult Considerations:* **,***	Take before bedtime. May be reduced after 1 to 2 nights.

*Take medication at bedtime.
**Start at the lowest dosage and titrate slowly while monitoring the patient for any side effects. Use lowest possible effective dose.
***Avoid in older adults; refer to Beers Criteria.
FDA, U.S. Food and Drug Administration.

Medication Side Effects

Common Side Effects

- Daytime drowsiness or sedation
- Increased fall risk/balance problems
- Mental slowing
- Orthostatic hypotension
- Unusual dreams
- Impaired driving
- Increased accidents due to sleepiness

Less Common Side Effects

- Attention difficulties
- Changes in appetite

Table 11.4

FDA-Approved Nonbenzodiazepines Dosage for Insomnia

Generic Name (Brand Name)	Dosage Forms	FDA Approval	Clinical Considerations
Eszopiclone (Lunesta)	Tablets	*Adults:* insomnia *Non-FDA Uses:* polysomnography, GAD (insomnia related), MDD (insomnia related), menopause (insomnia related) *Pediatrics:* safety in pediatric use has not been established *Older Adult Considerations*: *,**,***	Taken before bedtime. Advise patients to take tablets prior to at least 7 to 8 hours of sleep. Higher doses known to cause drowsiness and impairment on the following morning.
Zaleplon (Sonata)	Capsules	*Adults:* insomnia (short-term) *Pediatrics:* safety in pediatric use has not been established *Older Adult Considerations*: *,**,***	Taken before bedtime. Advise patients to take tablets prior to at least 7 to 8 hours of sleep.
Zolpidem (Ambien, Intermezzo, Edluar, Zolpimist, Sublinox)	*Tablets* (Ambien) *ER Tablets* (Ambien CR *Sublingual Tablets* (Edular) (Intermezzo) *Oral Spray* (Zolpimist)	*Adults:* insomnia (sleep onset and middle of night awakening) *Non-FDA Uses*: long-term insomnia, SSRI-induced insomnia *Pediatrics:* safety in pediatric use has not been established *Older Adult Considerations*: Use with Caution in older adults with dementia***	For Ambien tablets, Edular sublingual tablets, and Zolpimist oral spray, take before bedtime. For Intermezzo sublingual tablets, take before bedtime. Advise patients to take immediate-release tablets prior to at least 7 to 8 hours of sleep. Advise patients to take extended-release after awakening in the middle of the night when returning to sleep is difficult.

*Take medication at bedtime.
**Start at the lowest dosage and titrate slowly while monitoring the patient for any side effects.
***Avoid in older adults with dementia, delirium, or history of falls and/or fractures (Beers Criteria).
ER, extended release; FDA, U.S. Food and Drug Administration; GAD, generalized anxiety disorder; MDD, major depressive disorder; SSRI, selective serotonin reuptake inhibitor

- Constipation or diarrhea
- Dry mouth
- Dizziness
- Hallucinations
- Headache

Table 11.5

Sleep Therapy Approaches

Therapy	Key Features
Cognitive behavioral therapy for insomnia	▪ First-line and gold-standard intervention for insomnia ▪ Aims to change thought patterns that may be affecting sleep ▪ Efficacious in the short- and long-term management of insomnia ▪ Superior to pharmacotherapy in several randomized controlled trials (Mellor et al., 2019)
Relaxation training	▪ Techniques to promote physical and mental relaxation and reduce physical and thought processes that are negatively affecting sleep ▪ Progressive muscle relaxation: tensing groups of muscles of the body and then consciously relaxing them ▪ Autogenic training: involves focusing awareness on different parts of the body and consciously relaxing them ▪ Monitors measurements on a screen of how muscle relaxation or how certain thoughts affect each other
Biofeedback	▪ A method to feel how the body reacts to tensing and relaxing that involves placing electrodes on the body to measure muscle tension and pulse and brain activity
Bright light therapy	▪ Manages circadian rhythm disorders and gradually shifts sleep and wake times ▪ A lamp at 10,000 lux, portable visor light, or natural light exposure directly into the retina for 30 to 90 minutes immediately after waking from slee ▪ Improves daytime performance, alertness, and mood

NONPHARMACOLOGIC INTERVENTIONS

Sleep hygiene refers to a set of recommendations for the promotion of healthy sleep that includes behavioral and environmental components. Overall, individuals should obtain at least 7 hours of restful sleep each night. The following are common sleep hygiene recommendations.

Avoid/Limiting

- Limit consumption of food and drinks before bed; limit intake of caffeine after noon meal.
- Note patients use a light box with a light intensity measuring 10,000 lux[2], positioned between 16 to 24 inches away from the face.
- Establish a relaxing sleep environment.
- Avoid medications that disrupt sleep patterns; avoid alcohol.
- Go to bed at the same time each night.
- Have 30 to 45 minutes of quiet time before going to bed.
- Avoid overly stimulating activities before bedtime; avoid watching television; avoid using the phone while in bed.

Establishing a Sleep Environment

- Write down thoughts instead of ruminating on them while in bed.
- Listen to relaxing music/meditations to aid falling asleep.
- Remove clocks, telephones, and televisions from the bedroom.

Establishing a Sleep Schedule

- Regularly participate in physical activity during the morning or daytime.
- Stop exposure to light around 8 p.m.
- Note that light should shine into the patient's eyes indirectly, not directly.
- Set a timer to turn off the television once asleep.
- Make it a basic rule to only go to bed when feeling tired.

Essential Facts

In older adults, sleep disorders and depression are common, and in-light therapy has shown to be effective in treating these disorders (Sloane et al., 2008).

Essential Facts

Endogenous melatonin is secreted by the pineal gland during periods of darkness.

MAINTENANCE PHASE OF TREATMENT

Clinicians should provide ongoing education to patients that includes the pathophysiology, risk factors, natural history, clinical consequences, treatment options, any associated risks and/or conditions, and the patient's expectations. A specific follow-up plan and time frame should be outlined with the patient for the evaluation to be accurate and treatment options to be adjusted. General education on the impact of sleep hygiene, weight loss, sleep position, alcohol avoidance, risk-factor modification, and medication effects should be provided. If other specialists are involved in the patient's insomnia management, the sleep education should be delivered as part of a multidisciplinary management team.

CRITERIA FOR REFERRAL

Most patients with sleep problems are managed in primary-care settings. Due to time restraints, limited knowledge of sleep disorders medicine, high costs, and the limited number of specialty sleep centers, individuals with sleep problems receive suboptimal sleep-problem management in primary-care settings (Edinger et al., 2016). Appropriate and timely sleep referrals provide better overall patient care and improve health outcomes of patients.

Primary-care clinicians should refer the patient to a specialist under the following circumstances:

- The patient has experienced a long duration of insomnia without notable improvements.
- The patient experiences excessive daytime sleepiness where symptoms significantly impact daytime functioning, including the following:
  - Disturbed or restless sleep
  - Epworth Sleepiness Scale greater than or equal to 10
  - Fragmented sleep
  - Frequent unexplained arousals from sleep
  - Nonrestorative sleep or excessive fatigue
- The patient is at high risk for or provides evidence suggestive of disordered breathing. Risk factors and evidence include the following:
  - Apneas or hypoxemia during procedures requiring anesthesia
  - Choking or gasping during sleep
  - Cognitive deficits such as inattention or memory problems
  - Elongated/enlarged uvula
  - Erectile dysfunction
  - Habitual loud snoring
  - Heart conditions (congestive heart failure, atrial fibrillation, treatment refractory hypertension, nocturnal dysrhythmias, pulmonary hypertension)
  - High-arched/narrow hard palate
  - High-risk driving populations (commercial truck drivers)
  - Lateral peritonsillar narrowing
  - Morning headaches
  - Nasal abnormalities (polyps, deviation, valve abnormalities, turbinate hypertrophy).
  - Neck circumference greater than 17 inches in men or greater than 16 inches in women
  - Obesity or body mass index (BMI) greater than or equal to 30
  - Presence of retrognathia
  - Sleep-related bruxism
  - Stroke
  - Tonsillar hypertrophy
  - Type 2 diabetes
  - Unexplained nocturnal reflux
- Evidence suggests restless legs syndrome or periodic leg movement disorder.
- The patient requires sedative hypnotics for insomnia daily or on most days for 30 days or more.
- The presence of comorbid medical conditions is a key sign.

Patients should be referred to a psychiatrist if they are struggling with substance abuse or a severe concomitant mental health condition.

SUMMARY

Sleep conditions must be carefully considered in primary care. Insufficient sleep and resulting fatigue compromise personal safety and daytime performance and can negatively impact an individual's overall quality of life. Clinicians must be mindful that there is no "one size fits all" in the management of insomnia or other sleep-related conditions; therefore, patient-centered approaches are essential to optimal clinical outcomes.

RESOURCES

- American Academy of Sleep Medicine: https://aasm.org/clinical-resources/practice-standards/practice-guidelines
- Centers for Disease Control and Prevention: Sleep and sleep disorders
- Agency for Healthcare Research and Quality: Management of insomnia disorder in adults: Current state of the evidence
- 2017 American Academy of Sleep Medicine: Clinical practice guideline for the pharmacologic treatment of chronic insomnia in adults
- 2016 American College of Physicians: Management of insomnia in adults
- Clinical guideline for the treatment of primary insomnia

REVIEW QUESTIONS

1. During which one of the following stages of sleep does dreaming occur?
   a. Nonrapid eye movement sleep (NREM) stage
   b. Rapid eye movement (REM) sleep stage
   c. Wakefulness stage before the NREM sleep stages and REM sleep stages begin
   d. In between NREM sleep and REM sleep
2. During periods of darkness, which one of the following glands in the brain helps to regulate circadian rhythms and releases the hormone melatonin?
   a. Pineal gland
   b. Pituitary gland
   c. Hypothalamus gland
   d. Parathyroid gland
3. First-line treatment and the gold-standard intervention in the management of insomnia is which one of the following?
   a. Bright light therapy
   b. Relaxation therapy
   c. Cognitive behavioral therapy for insomnia
   d. Biofeedback
4. Which one of the following statements is false?
   a. The most diagnosed sleep disorder is insomnia.
   b. Sleep hygiene is a method that promotes healthy sleep using behavioral and environmental components.

c. Insufficient sleep and daytime sleepiness can compromise a person's safety and performance and negatively impact their overall quality of life.
d. In older adults, use of benzodiazepines does not need to be avoided in the treatment of insomnia if they are prescribed in low doses.

5. Which one of the following statements is the most accurate?
   a. Factors that have been shown to influence circadian rhythm disruptions do not include emotional, behavioral, genetic, or environmental influences, but have shown to be primarily influenced by melatonin production.
   b. Poor sleep has shown to not be associated with increased rates of morbidity and mortality.
   c. Treatment goals in the management of insomnia include the improvement of sleep quality, sleep duration, sleep satisfaction, and reducing daytime impairments caused by excessive daytime sleepiness.
   d. None of the above are accurate statements.

REFERENCES

American Psychiatric Association. (2013). *Diagnostic and statistical manual of mental disorders* (5th ed.). https://doi.org/10.1176/appi.books.9780890425596

Buysse, D. J. (2014). Sleep health: Can we define it? Does it matter? *Sleep, 37*(1), 9–17. https://doi.org/10.5665/sleep.3298

Cormier, R. E. (1990). Sleep disturbances. In Walker, H. K., Hall, W. D., & Hurst, J. W. (Eds.), *Clinical methods: The history, physical, and laboratory examinations*, (3rd ed., pp. 398–403). Butterworths.

Edinger, J. D., Grubber, J., Ulmer, C., Zervakis, J., & Olsen, M. (2016). A collaborative paradigm for improving management of sleep disorders in primary care: A randomized clinical trial. *Sleep, 39*(1), 237–247. https://doi.org/10.5665/sleep.5356

Freeman, D., Sheaves, B., Goodwin, G. M., Yu, L. M., Nickless, A., Harrison, P. J., Emsley, R., Luik, A. I., Foster, R. G., Wadekar, V., Hinds, C., Gumley, A., Jones, R., Lightman, S., Jones, S., Bentall, R., Kinderman, P., Rowse, G., Brugha, T., … Espie, C. A. (2017). The effects of improving sleep on mental health (OASIS): A randomised controlled trial with mediation analysis. *The Lancet Psychiatry, 4*(10), 749–758. https://doi.org/10.1016/S2215-0366(17)30328-0

Huang, H., Zhang, J., Zhu, L., Tang, J., Lin, G., Kong, W., Lei, X., & Zhu, L. (2021). EEG-based sleep staging analysis with functional connectivity. *Sensors, 21*(6), Article 1988. https://doi.org/10.3390/s21061988

Kapur, V. K., Auckley, D. H., Chowdhuri, S., Kuhlmann, D. C., Mehra, R., Ramar, K., & Harrod, C. G. (2017). Clinical practice guideline for diagnostic testing for adult obstructive sleep apnea: An American Academy of Sleep Medicine clinical practice guideline. *Journal of Clinical Sleep Medicine, 13*(3), 479–504. https://doi.org/10.5664/jcsm.6506

Krystal, A. D. (2015). New developments in insomnia medications of relevance to mental health disorders. *The Psychiatric Clinics of North America, 38*(4), 843–860. https://doi.org/10.1016/j.psc.2015.08.001

Mead, M. P., & Irish, L. A. (2020). Application of health behaviour theory to sleep health improvement. *Journal of Sleep Research, 29*(5), Article e12950. https://doi.org/10.1111/jsr.12950

Mellor, A., Hamill, K., Jenkins, M. M., Baucom, D. H., Norton, P. J., & Drummond, S. (2019). Partner-assisted cognitive behavioural therapy for insomnia versus cognitive behavioural therapy for insomnia: A randomised controlled trial. *Trials*, *20*(1), Article 262. https://doi.org/10.1186/s13063-019-3334-3

Rezaie, L., Maazinezhad, S., Fogelberg, D. J., Khazaie, H., Sadeghi-Bahmani, D., & Brand, S. (2021). Compared to individuals with mild to moderate obstructive sleep apnea (OSA), individuals with severe OSA had higher BMI and respiratory-disturbance scores. *Life*, *11*(5), Article 368. https://doi.org/10.3390/life11050368

Sateia, M. J., Buysse, D. J., Krystal, A. D., Neubauer, D. N., & Heald, J. L. (2017). Clinical practice guideline for the pharmacologic treatment of chronic insomnia in adults: An American Academy of Sleep Medicine clinical practice guideline. *Journal of Clinical Sleep Medicine*, *13*(2), 307–349. https://doi.org/10.5664/jcsm.6470

Seow, L., Verma, S. K., Mok, Y. M., Kumar, S., Chang, S., Satghare, P., Hombali, A., Vaingankar, J., Chong, S. A., & Subramaniam, M. (2018). Evaluating *DSM-5* insomnia disorder and the treatment of sleep problems in a psychiatric population. *Journal of Clinical Sleep Medicine*, *14*(2), 237–244. https://doi.org/10.5664/jcsm.6942

Slavish, D. C., Taylor, D. J., & Lichstein, K. L. (2019). Intraindividual variability in sleep and comorbid medical and mental health conditions. *Sleep*, *42*(6), Article zsz052. https://doi.org/10.1093/sleep/zsz052

Sloane, P. D., Figueiro, M., & Cohen, L. (2008). Light as therapy for sleep disorders and depression in older adults. *Clinical Geriatrics*, *16*(3), 25–31. https://www.ncbi.nlm.nih.gov/pmc/articles/PMC3839957

Watson, N. F., Badr, M. S., Belenky, G., Bliwise, D. L., Buxton, O. M., Buysse, D., Dinges, D. F., Gangwisch, J., Grandner, M. A., Kushida, C., Malhotra, R. K., Martin, J. L., Patel, S. R., Quan, S. F., & Tasali, E. (2015). Recommended amount of sleep for a healthy adult: A joint consensus statement of the American Academy of Sleep Medicine and Sleep Research Society. *Sleep*, *38*(6), 843–844. https://doi.org/10.5665/sleep.4716

Worley, S. L. (2018). The extraordinary importance of sleep: The detrimental effects of inadequate sleep on health and public safety drive an explosion of sleep research. *Pharmacy and Therapeutics*, *43*(12), 758–763. https://www.ncbi.nlm.nih.gov/pmc/articles/PMC6281147

III

Nonmedication Treatments

12

Nonmedication Treatments

Psychologic interventions include a broad range of treatment possibilities that aim to modify behaviors, emotions, or feelings to maximize an individual's overall functioning and well-being. Psychologic interventions can be delivered to an individual, a group, or a combination of both. The National Institute of Health and Care Excellence guidelines discuss the evidence and the role of psychologic interventions for improving clinical outcomes in individuals with mental health conditions and consider the distinct needs of individuals and their families. Encouraging strong family, caregiver, and school partnerships that include coordinating efforts and help with management may enhance the effects of psychosocial treatments.

In this chapter you will learn:

1. Which psychotherapy interventions are used to treat and manage mental health conditions
2. Which nonmedication treatment options can be used in the management of mental health
3. How to name five key features of cognitive behavioral therapy
4. How to identify the goals of psychoeducation for individuals, families, couples, and groups
5. How to incorporate diet and exercise into management plans for optimal therapeutic responses in mental health conditions

Different strategies can be used to manage mild, moderate, and severe affective, cognitive, and behavioral symptoms. Although some individuals with severe symptoms may require medications, psychotherapy, natural supplements, and lifestyle changes to feel better and optimize their functioning, others with mild or moderately severe symptoms may respond well to lifestyle changes alone and require ongoing encouragement to engage in consistent positive lifestyle changes before taking a psychotropic medication. Although numerous psychologic interventions have been shown to be effective, this chapter specifically discusses psychoeducation, psychotherapy, cognitive behavioral therapy, exercise, and diet.

PSYCHOEDUCATION

To foster a supportive and empathetic environment, clinicians must (a) provide patients and families with safe and structured education, counseling, and resources; and (b) teach communication skills and coping skills to those with different cultural backgrounds and different psychiatric disorders. Psychoeducation, an evidence-based practice, has been shown to significantly reduce relapse and hospitalization among individuals with various mental health conditions and decrease the burden and stress levels of caregivers (Varghese et al., 2020). Psychoeducation involves equipping patients with education and therapeutic techniques by providing basic information about the patient's illness and the illness's course, causes, treatment, and prognosis (Yatham et al., 2018). Patients must be provided time to grasp the information that may be unfamiliar and challenging, and clinicians should provide the available resources for support of a particular illness (Zhao et al., 2015).

Table 12.1 lists the goals of psychotherapy. Informative sessions can be delivered in face-to-face interactions with a practitioner. Additionally, informative sessions that involve online tools, smartphone apps, and workbooks are currently being tested (Yatham et al., 2018). Sessions can vary in length depending on the time available with clients and their caregivers, and sessions typically occur during medical appointments and therapy sessions. Often, individuals with mental illness have little to no insight regarding the presence of their illness, making it difficult for caregivers to cope.

Table 12.1

Goals of Psychoeducation

Key information on the diagnosed condition and challenges	▪ Name of condition ▪ Symptoms of the condition ▪ Cause of the condition (genetic, biologic, environmental) ▪ Condition management
Treatment options	▪ Medications (how they work, restrictions or possible risks, effects on the body) ▪ Lifestyle changes ▪ Self-help options to relieve discomfort and pain
Problem-solving skills	▪ Identify problems ▪ Identify those affected by the problem ▪ Learn to assess options and get further information (videos, handout, ask questions) ▪ Evaluate treatment options and solutions

PSYCHOTHERAPY

Psychotherapy, also referred to as talk therapy, is an evidence-based, structured, therapeutic framework based on psychologic principles that are used to help individuals with a broad variety of mental illnesses and emotional difficulties eliminate, reduce, or control troubling symptoms. In other words, psychotherapy enables a person to function optimally and increases their well-being. Psychotherapy can be delivered in different formats, and no one approach is better than another; often, blended approaches are effective. Table 12.2 provides the key features of the different formats of psychotherapy.

Psychotherapy has been shown to reduce patients' severity of symptoms and suicidality and may reduce self-harm and mood dysregulation while improving psychosocial functioning. Cuijpers et al. (2014) conducted a meta-analysis of studies comparing pharmacotherapy alone with combined pharmacotherapy and psychotherapy. The authors found that pharmacotherapy and psychotherapy interventions are largely independent of each other and provide additive benefits. They do not interfere with each other, and both contribute about equally to positive treatment outcomes. According to Dunlop (2016), combination treatment during acute and continuation phases may increase remission rates, shorten the time required to achieve remission, and enhance adherence to treatment.

Table 12.2

Formats for Psychotherapy Delivery

Format	Key Features
Individual	■ A confidential joint process between a clinician and patient receiving therapy ■ Goals of therapy are to inspire change, overcome obstacles, increase positive feelings, learn coping styles, reach goals, or improve quality of life
Group	■ One or more clinicians and two or more patients receiving therapy that offers supportive networks for people who have similar difficulties ■ A group of individuals that can instill hope and promote interpersonal learning and socializing techniques ■ Sharing of emotions and perspectives among group members
Family	■ Designed to address specific issues that affect a family and find solutions to problems and ways to work together as a unit
Couple	■ Couples involved in a romantic relationship meet with a clinician to gain insight into their relationship, resolve conflict, and improve relationship satisfaction
Computerized platforms and mobile apps	■ Both as self-directed and therapist-guided ■ Innovation in mental health apps to ultimately deliver large-scale impact on public health ■ Mobile apps can enhance psychoeducation ■ Mobile interventions that also incorporate symptom tracking ■ Support in-the-moment self-assessments

Typically, psychologic therapies are based on assumptions about causality, core symptoms, and maintenance of the disorder. There are hundreds of psychotherapeutic approaches and different ways to categorize them; many approaches have existed for years, and new methods continue to emerge. According to Humer et al. (2020), therapy approaches can be broadly categorized into four general themes: (a) behavioral, (b) humanistic, (c), psychodynamic, and (d) systemic. Table 12.3 provides an overview of the four styles. Other common approaches include cognitive behavioral therapy (CBT), dialectical behavior therapy, hypnotherapy, interpersonal psychotherapy, solution-focused therapy, supportive individual and group therapy, motivational interviewing, couple and family therapy, mindfulness-based therapy (MBT), self-help programs (SHPs), phone- and internet-based therapies, remote videoconferencing, and other health interventions (e.g., smartphone apps). See the following Essentials box for details on the role of the clinician during therapy sessions.

Essential Facts

Essential Roles of the Therapy Clinician

- High priority is given to self-harm and suicidal behaviors.
- Maintain the therapeutic relationship:
  - affect regulation
  - tolerance of emotional states
  - biases in social cognition
- Offer explorative and change-oriented interventions.
- Assess options for treatment formats (e.g., includes both individual and group therapy).
- Provide support and validation.
- Consider psychoeducation

Table 12.3

Key Features of Psychotherapy Approaches

Psychotherapies	Key Features
Behavioral therapy	Relies on behavioral techniques for transformation of maladaptive patterns of behavior or thoughts to improve emotional responses, reactions, and behaviors
Humanistic or "experiential" therapy	Derived from humanistic psychology Focuses on human development and individual needs while highlighting growth and subjective meaning
Psychodynamic therapy	Centered on revealing or interpreting unconscious conflicts
Systemic therapy	Emphasis on interactions, patterns, and dynamics of groups rather than on the individual Looks to identify distinct patterns of group behaviors (e.g., families)

COGNITIVE BEHAVIORAL THERAPY

CBT, founded by psychologists Albert Eilis and Aaron T. Beck (Dunlop, 2016), is considered one of the most common and best studied forms of psychotherapy. CBT is based on the idea that the way people think (cognition), feel (emotion), and act (behavior) relate to each other. CBT is a type of psychotherapy that combines two therapeutic approaches: cognitive therapy and behavioral therapy. The behavioral aspect of CBT is based on the premise that changing behavior leads to changing emotion and cognition; however, the cognitive feature centers on changing cognition, which is thought to change emotion and behavior (Kaczkurkin & Foa, 2015).

CBT is a skill-focused, psychotherapeutic framework that helps individuals identify and change maladaptive, destructive, or disturbing thought patterns that can trigger negative behavioral and emotional responses. Some of the methods used in CBT include challenging one's automatic negative thoughts to then change one's underlying beliefs that negatively impact thought processes. Behavioral strategies include self-monitoring, scheduling daily activities, rating pleasure and accomplishment with activities, and role-playing to reinforce the relationship between an individual's actions and mood and to encourage positive behaviors that align with long-term goals.

CBT is used to treat a wide variety of physical and mental health conditions, such as anxiety, depression, obsessive-compulsive disorder, posttraumatic stress disorder (PTSD), social phobias, sleep disturbances, substance dependence, chronic pain, and more. Relaxation exercises, stress- and pain-relief methods, and problem-solving strategies can also be incorporated into CBT sessions and can help improve stress, worry, mood, or emotional well-being. Homework prescribed by practitioners can be an integral component of CBT because homework allows patients to practice and reinforce the skills learned in therapy sessions in real life. Homework can include (a) psychoeducational homework, (b) self-assessment homework, and (c) modality-specific homework (Tang & Kreindler, 2017). Examples of homework assignments are symptom logs, self-reflective journals, specific structured activities like exposure and response prevention for obsessions and compulsions, and monitoring one's mood using thought records. According to Tang and Kreindler (2017), CBT homework can be described as specific, structured, therapeutic activities that are routinely discussed in session and are to be completed between sessions.

Essential Facts

CBT is a goal-directed type of psychotherapy that encourages new ways of thinking and offers new skills and strategies for overcoming problems. It also focuses on personal development and prevention of relapse.

EXERCISE

The integration of physical activity interventions for individuals with mental health problems can promote recovery and reduce the mental, physical, and social burden and disability associated with mental health conditions. Lifestyle modifications are essential to physical and mental health. An essential part of lifestyle modification includes physical activity and exercise, which are often referred to as modifiable risk factors. According to Stanton et al. (2019), individuals with severe mental illness are 3.5 times more likely to experience fatal conditions due to the strong association between mental health and cardiovascular diseases. Evidence suggests that exercise may have similar benefits to pharmacologic interventions with respect to (a) reducing mortality in people with cardiovascular disease and depression, (b) establishing an earlier onset of recovery, (c) increasing remission rates, and (d) lowering relapse rates. According to Lattari et al. (2018), studies have shown that aerobic physical activity has acute anxiolytic and antipanic effects among individuals with panic disorders. Additionally, physical activity and exercise have been shown to benefit cardiac health among people with depression and anxiety (Yatham et al., 2018). Physical activity such as aerobic exercise has been studied and validated for reducing symptoms and treating anxiety, depression, eating disorders, bipolar disorders, schizophrenia, addictions, grief, relationship problems, dementia, personality disorders, and a variety of other mental conditions (National Institute of Health and Care Excellence, 2009; Rethorst et al., 2009). According to Sharma et al. (2006), exercise increases blood circulation to the brain and has an influence on the hypothalamic-pituitary-adrenal (HPA) axis, which elicits a stress response. Furthermore, exercise can (a) increase levels of serotonin, dopamine, norepinephrine, and endorphins; (b) balance neurotransmitter levels in the brain; and (c) elevate mood.

Essential Facts

Physical activity can alter the gut microbiome and promote microbial diversity to help fight against gastrointestinal disorders, increase immune responses, and reduce obesity (Monda et al., 2017).

Essential Facts

Benefits of Exercise on Mental and Physical Health

The following are the benefits of exercise on mental and physical health:

- Deepens relaxation.
- Enhances mood.
- Helps balance neurotransmitter levels.
- Improves blood glucose levels.
- Improves blood pressure.
- Improves energy.
- Improves mental clarity, learning, insight, memory, and cognitive functioning.

(*continued*)

Essential Facts (*continued*)

- Improves sleep.
- Improves social health and relationships.
- Increases levels of serotonin, dopamine, and norepinephrine.
- Prevents cardiac disease.
- Raises self-esteem and increases spiritual connection.
- Reduces cholesterol.
- Reduces stress.
- Strengthens muscle and bone.

GOAL-SETTING OBJECTIVES

Table 12.4 provides a goal-setting framework using specific, measurable, attainable, relevant, and timely (SMART) goals for personal improvement. SMART goals can be used to help clients track their progress and alter their plans when necessary.

Other important factors to consider when integrating physical activity and exercise to manage mental healthcare include the following:

- Start with what patients know and work from there (assess health literacy).
- Assess readiness for change.
- Identify barriers to change.
- Start with small changes in a patient's life and do not insist on an overhaul.
- Using simple and clear language, explain the rationale for the treatment.
- Use culturally sensitive approaches (inquire about beliefs and interpretations about behavior change).

Table 12.4

SMART Goal-Setting Objectives

Goal-Setting Objectives	Key Features
Specific	Include details like who, what, when, where, and why. For example, "I will walk on my treadmill for 30 minutes five times per week because it is good for my physical and mental health."
Measurable	Is a quantity associated with the goal to evaluate progress? For example, how many minutes of exercise and how often during a week?
Attainable	Assess that goal attainment is reasonable. Is it realistic? For example, how realistic is this goal given the patient's schedule? What would be a more attainable goal?
Relevant	Assessment of goal relevance to the patient. Why is exercise relevant to the patient? How will this change improve the patient's life?
Timely	Define a specific timeline for the goal. When will the goal be achieved? Is it a short-term or long-term goal? When will the follow-up appointment be scheduled?

- Provide a consistent, warm, and positive environment to promote questions and voicing of concerns.
- Check with practitioner before initiating exercise.
- Engage with patient without judgment.
- Help establish goals, desired outcomes, and reasons for change.
- Plan detailed goals to ensure that goals are SMART.
- Identify resources needed to achieve goals.
- Keep a record of physical activity and exercise.
- Set up evaluation method to assess plan.

DIETARY PATTERNS, GUT HEALTH, AND MENTAL HEALTH

Nutritional psychiatry is an emerging field that aims to investigate how dietary patterns, diet quality, and dietary components impact mental and sleep health. Nutrition has been linked to behavior, mood, and the pathology and treatment of mental illness. Studies have shown that due to the communication between the gut–brain axis, a healthy diet promotes a healthy gut; therefore, various nutrients, nutritional deficiencies or abundancies, food items, diet quality, and diet type may impact mental health and sleep (Hepsomali & Groeger, 2021). Large population studies have found that people who eat a lot of nutrient-dense foods report less depression and superior levels of happiness and mental well-being (Moreno-Agostino et al., 2019).

Gut microbiota are involved in the body's protective functions and in the maintenance of its homeostasis and are influenced by stress, emotion, pain, and various neurotransmitters. The human gastrointestinal tract contains approximately 1,014 microorganisms, and their genome—the microbiome—originates from about 1,000 to 1,150 bacterial species; it contains a gene set approximately 150 times greater than that of the human genome (Monda et al., 2017). Strong evidence suggests that gut microbiota produce neurochemicals that influence the peripheral enteric and central nervous systems, which has led to the microbiota-gut–brain axis' being identified as the primary nutrient-mediated pathway involved in the regulation of mental health (Carabotti et al., 2015). The role of the gut–brain axis is to monitor and connect gut functions to emotional and cognitive brain regions with peripheral intestinal functions and mechanisms, such as immune activation, intestinal permeability, enteric reflex, and entero-endocrine signaling (Carabotti et al., 2015). The gastrointestinal tract is where billions of bacteria are produced, and these bacteria influence the production of serotonin, dopamine, and other neurotransmitters involved in delivering messages from the gut to the brain. Foods that are high in sugar can induce inflammatory processes and hamper neurotransmitter production. For example, consuming nutritious and healthy foods promotes the growth of bacteria that positively affect neurotransmitter production. In their review of 56 studies, Khanna et al. (2019) found an association between a high intake of Mediterranean diet foods such as olive oil, fish, nuts, legumes, dairy products, fruits, and vegetables and a reduced risk of depression during adolescence. However, western diets that include the consumption of sweetened beverages high in sugar, fried foods high in fat, processed meats, and baked products were associated with an increased risk of depression in longitudinal studies (Khanna et al., 2019).

Serotonin helps regulate sleep, appetite, pain, and mood. Serotonin is produced in the gastrointestinal tract, which is linked with millions of nerve cells and helps to control one's emotions. The bacteria and chemicals that make up the intestinal microbiota can regulate nerve signals (the vagus nerve is the primary connection between the brain and intestinal tract) and alter neurotransmitter levels in the brain. These molecules, which are secreted by the digestive system, can affect brain function, including sleep, appetite, mood, and cognition. Because the gut communicates with cells throughout the human body, it is often referred to as the body's *second brain*.

Essential Facts

Dysbiosis, the imbalance of flora in the gut microbiome, can be caused by chronic stress, environmental toxins, cigarette smoke, alcohol, medications, malnutrition (diet), genetics, infections, chronic illnesses, allergies, poor sleep and chronic fatigue, and lack of physical activity.

EFFECTS OF FOOD ON MEDICATION BIOAVAILABILITY

Food intake can influence the bioavailability of certain psychotropic drugs. Food may interfere with how medications pass through the gastrointestinal tract and the metabolic transformation of drugs in the gastrointestinal wall and in the liver. Ingested food products may also interfere with how the drug is broken down in the body. An astute nurse practitioner will inquire about medications, herbal supplements, over-the-counter medications, and diet to acquire the information needed to educate patients on best practices for maximum medication absorption. Table 12.5 provides general information on commonly consumed foods and lifestyle behaviors that influence the pharmacokinetic interaction with drugs.

Essential Facts

Rates of tobacco smoking are higher among individuals with psychiatric illness than in the general population. Smoking rates are estimated to be two to five times higher in individuals with schizophrenia, mood disorders, anxiety disorders, attention deficit hyperactivity disorder, binge-eating disorder, bulimia, and substance use disorders (Boksa, 2017).

There is no one-size-fits-all lifestyle approach; therefore, it is important to consider each patient's distinct needs, take a patient-centered approach to treatment, and consider the targeted disease, the patient's culture, the sustainability of the patient's diet, and the patient's available resources.

Table 12.5

Diet and Lifestyle Behaviors That Influence the Pharmacokinetic Interaction With Drugs

Diet and Lifestyle Behaviors	Key Features
Vitamin C (ascorbic acid)	■ Urine excretion increases if stimulants (amphetamine, lisdexamfetamine) are taken with foods or drinks that are high in ascorbic acid ■ May decrease blood levels of medication ■ Vitamin C does not affect the rate of methylphenidate excretion
Grapefruit juice	■ Inhibits the CYP450 3A4 isoforms ■ Contains bioflavonoids that raise bioavailability concentrations (anxiolytics, antidepressants, mood stabilizers, antipsychotics, and procognitive compounds)
Caffeine	■ 90% of adults in the United States consume caffeine (Belayneh & Molla, 2020) ■ Inhibits the cytochrome CYP450 1A2 pathway; therefore, caffeine and drugs act as a metabolic inhibitor to each other and can decrease the rate of their elimination ■ Alters dissolution profile, gastrointestinal pH, gastrointestinal emptying time, and the formation of inhibiting glucose-6-phosphatase ■ Inhibits vitamin D, zinc, and calcium absorption ■ Although highly variable, caffeine can inhibit or decrease absorption of neuroleptic drugs (phenothiazines, clozapine), lithium, theophylline, warfarin, zolpidem, and several antidepressants and antipsychotic drugs (Belayneh & Molla, 2020) ■ Cutting back on coffee decreases serum clozapine levels; intake of coffee inhibits 1A2 and increases clozapine blood levels ■ May induce or accelerate absorption rates for aspirin, ergotamine, levodopa
Smoking	■ Induces hepatic CYP450 1A2 drug-metabolizing enzymes ■ Induces the metabolism of psychotropic drugs, including the antipsychotics clozapine and olanzapine, and other agents, such as other antipsychotics and benzodiazepines ■ Mean plasma levels of clozapine are lower in smokers than nonsmokers, and in a patient quitting smoking, clozapine levels are predicted to rise within 1 to 2 days after smoking cessation (Boksa, 2017)
Charcoal-grilled meat and broccoli (consumed for longer than 5 days)	■ Induces CYP1A2 activity ■ Increases metabolism of caffeine (i.e., CYP1A probe) ■ Clozapine, olanzapine, and duloxetine are partially metabolized by CYP1A2 and can therefore result in decreased drug exposure

FOODS THAT PROMOTE MENTAL WELLNESS

The following foods promote mental wellness:

- Antioxidants (dark chocolate, blueberries, strawberries)
- Colorful, fresh fruits and vegetables
- Fermented foods (sauerkraut, kefir, tempe)
- Fiber (pears, avocados, apples)
- Fish
- Folate (beans, lentils)
- Fresh foods (organic, non-GMO)
- Lean meats
- Magnesium (dark chocolate, nuts and seeds, legumes, spinach)
- Plant proteins (beans, legumes)
- Vitamin D (salmon, portabella mushrooms, yogurt, milk)
- Whole foods (not fragmented, refined, or processed)

Essential Facts

Food optimizes the absorption of some psychotropic drugs, including ziprasidone, vilazodone, and lurasidone.

Essential Facts

According to the World Health Organization (2004), good mental health is a "state of well-being in which the individual realizes his or her own abilities, can cope with the normal stresses of life, can work productively and fruitfully, and is able to make a contribution to his or her community" (para 1).

SUMMARY

Psychoeducation, psychotherapy, physical activity, and nutritional counseling are crucial to optimal mental and physical health, functioning, and wellness. Physical activity and dietary patterns are instrumental for robust immune responses, modulation of inflammation, and prevention and management of chronic disease. Clinicians should continuously inquire about changes in patients' lifestyle behaviors, such as caffeine intake and smoking habits, due to these behaviors' influence on psychotropic medications. Through effective communication, psychoeducation enables clients to better understand how physical activity and gut health are linked to mental health and can help protect against disease, obesity, mood disorders, dementia, and many other conditions.

REVIEW QUESTIONS

1. Caffeine ______ CYP450 1A2 and _____ clozapine levels.
   a. Inhibits and increases
   b. Inhibits and decreases
   c. Decreases and stabilizes
   d. Increases and stabilizes
2. Which one of the following statements is false?
   a. High ascorbic acid (vitamin C) intake increases the excretion of amphetamines but does not impact methylphenidate.
   b. Caffeine inhibits CYP450 1A4 activity.
   c. Smoking induces CYP450 1A2 activity.
   d. Grapefruit juice induces the CYP450 3A4 isoforms due to bioflavonoids that lower bioavailability concentrations of psychotropic drugs.
3. The SMART acronym used for goal setting stands for which one of the following objectives?
   a. SMART is an acronym for specific, measurable, attainable, relevant, and timely goals.
   b. SMART is an acronym for standard, meaningful, actionable, rare, and theoretical goals.
   c. SMART is an acronym for specific, minute, alternative, relevant, and timely goals.
   d. SMART is an acronym for specific, measurable, attainable, relevant, and totality of goals.
4. Which one of the following best describes the purpose of psychoeducation?
   a. Psychoeducation provides the client, family, and/or caregivers with information about the illness; its course, causes, treatment, prognosis, and available supportive resources; and provides a response to questions or concerns.
   b. Psychoeducation provides therapy sessions using a skill-focused psychotherapeutic framework to help individuals identify and change maladaptive, destructive, or disturbing thought patterns that can trigger negative behavioral and emotional responses.
   c. Psychoeducation provides an educational process derived from humanistic psychology that focuses on human development and individual needs, while highlighting growth and subjective meaning.
   d. Psychoeducation is designed to address specific issues that affect family dynamics, to find solutions to problems and ways to work together as a unit, and to share where irrational thoughts can impact emotions and behaviors.
5. Which one of the following statements is the most accurate?
   a. Exercise decreases levels of serotonin, dopamine, norepinephrine, and endorphins and helps balance neurotransmitter levels in the brain and elevate mood.
   b. Psychoeducation, psychotherapy, physical activity, and dietary patterns are not highly associated with optimal mental and physical health and well-being because medication effects are more important.
   c. It is important to inquire about caffeine intake at each follow-up visit because caffeine alters the dissolution profile of psychotropic

medications, alters gastrointestinal pH, affects gastrointestinal emptying times, and impacts the formation of inhibiting glucose-6-phosphatase that can impact medication levels.

d. None of the above are accurate statements.

REFERENCES

Belayneh, A., & Molla, F. (2020). The effect of coffee on pharmacokinetic properties of drugs: A review. *BioMed Research International, 2020*, Article 7909703. https://doi.org/10.1155/2020/7909703

Boksa, P. (2017). Smoking, psychiatric illness and the brain. *Journal of Psychiatry & Neuroscience, 42*(3), 147–149. https://doi.org/10.1503/jpn.170060

Carabotti, M., Scirocco, A., Maselli, M. A., & Severi, C. (2015). The gut-brain axis: Interactions between enteric microbiota, central and enteric nervous systems. *Annals of Gastroenterology, 28*(2), 203–209. https://www.ncbi.nlm.nih.gov/pmc/articles/PMC4367209

Cuijpers, P., Sijbrandij, M., Koole, S. L., Andersson, G., Beekman, A. T., & Reynolds, C. F., III. (2014). Adding psychotherapy to antidepressant medication in depression and anxiety disorders: A meta-analysis. *World Psychiatry, 13*(1), 56–67. https://doi.org/10.1002/wps.20089

Dunlop, B. W. (2016). Evidence-based applications of combination psychotherapy and pharmacotherapy for depression. *Focus, 14*(2), 156–173. https://doi.org/10.1176/appi.focus.20150042

Hepsomali, P., & Groeger, J. A. (2021). Diet, sleep, and mental health: Insights from the UK Biobank Study. *Nutrients, 13*(8), Article 2573. https://doi.org/10.3390/nu13082573

Humer, E., Stippl, P., Pieh, C., Pryss, R., & Probst, T. (2020). Experiences of psychotherapists with remote psychotherapy during the COVID-19 pandemic: Cross-sectional web-based survey study. *Journal of Medical Internet Research, 22*(11), Article e20246. https://doi.org/10.2196/20246

Kaczkurkin, A. N., & Foa, E. B. (2015). Cognitive-behavioral therapy for anxiety disorders: An update on the empirical evidence. *Dialogues in Clinical Neuroscience, 17*(3), 337–346. https://doi.org/10.31887/DCNS.2015.17.3/akaczkurkin

Khanna, P., Chattu, V. K., & Aeri, B. T. (2019). Nutritional aspects of depression in adolescents—A systematic review. *International Journal of Preventive Medicine, 10*, Article 42. https://doi.org/10.4103/ijpvm.IJPVM_400_18

Lattari, E., Budde, H., Paes, F., Neto, G., Appolinario, J. C., Nardi, A. E., Murillo-Rodriguez, E., & Machado, S. (2018). Effects of aerobic exercise on anxiety symptoms and cortical activity in patients with panic disorder: A pilot study. *Clinical Practice and Epidemiology in Mental Health, 14*, 11–25. https://doi.org/10.2174/1745017901814010011

Monda, V., Villano, I., Messina, A., Valenzano, A., Esposito, T., Moscatelli, F., Viggiano, A., Cibelli, G., Chieffi, S., Monda, M., & Messina, G. (2017). Exercise modifies the gut microbiota with positive health effects. *Oxidative Medicine and Cellular Longevity*, 2017, Article 3831972. https://doi.org/10.1155/2017/3831972

Moreno-Agostino, D., Caballero, F. F., Martín-María, N., Tyrovolas, S., López-García, P., Rodríguez-Artalejo, F., Haro, J. P., Ayuso-Mateos, J. L., & Miret, M. (2019). Mediterranean diet and wellbeing: Evidence from a nationwide survey. *Psychology & Health, 34*(3), 321–335. https://doi.org/10.1080/08870446.2018.1525492

National Institute for Health and Care Excellence. (2009). *Depression in adults: Recognition and management.* from https://www.nice.org.uk/guidance/cg90

Rethorst, C. D., Wipfli, B. M., & Landers, D. M. (2009). The antidepressive effects of exercise: A meta-analysis of randomized trials. *Sports Medicine, 39*(6), 491–511. https://doi.org/10.2165/00007256-200939060-00004

Sharma, A., Madaan, V., & Petty, F. D. (2006). Exercise for mental health. *Primary Care Companion to the Journal of Clinical Psychiatry, 8*(2), Article 106. https://dx.doi.org/10.4088%2Fpcc.v08n0208a

Stanton, R., Rebar, A., & Rosenbaum, S. (2019). Exercise and mental health literacy in an Australian adult population. *Depression & Anxiety, 36*(5), 465–472. https://doi.org/10.1002/da.22851

Tang, W., & Kreindler, D. (2017). Supporting homework compliance in cognitive behavioural therapy: Essential features of mobile apps. *JMIR Mental Health, 4*(2), Article e20. https://doi.org/10.2196/mental.5283

Varghese, M., Kirpekar, V., & Loganathan, S. (2020). Family interventions: Basic principles and techniques. *Indian Journal of Psychiatry, 62*, S192–S200. https://doi.org/10.4103/psychiatry.IndianJPsychiatry_770_19

World Health Organization. (2004). *Prevention of mental disorders: Effective interventions and policy options.* https://apps.who.int/iris/handle/10665/43027

Yatham, L. N., Kennedy, S. H., Parikh, S. V., Schaffer, A., Bond, D. J., Frey, B. N., Sharma, V., Goldstein, B. I., Rej, S., Beaulieu, S., Alda, M., MacQueen, G., Milev, R. V., Ravindran, A., O'Donovan, C., McIntosh, D., Lam, R. W., Vazquez, G., Kapczinski, F., … Berk, M. (2018). Canadian Network for Mood and Anxiety Treatments (CANMAT) and International Society for Bipolar Disorders (ISBD) 2018 guidelines for the management of patients with bipolar disorder. *Bipolar Disorders, 20*(2), 97–170. https://doi.org/10.1111/bdi.12609

Zhao, S., Sampson, S., Xia, J., & Jayaram, M. B. (2015). Psychoeducation (brief) for people with serious mental illness. *Cochrane Database of Systematic Reviews, 4*, Article CD010823. https://doi.org/10.1002/14651858.cd010823.pub2

IV

Answers to Review Questions

13

Answers to Review Questions

CHAPTER 1: THE PSYCHIATRIC INTERVIEW

1. **c.** *Pharmacodynamics* is the study of a drug's molecular, biochemical, and physiologic effects or actions on the body.
2. **b.** The percentage of suicide attempts is 10 to 30 times higher than completed suicides.
3. **a.** *Reliability* refers to the consistency of a measure and the ability to reproduce results under equivalent conditions.
4. **b.** Promotion of self-management strategies is part of the termination phase.
5. **c.** *Sensitivity* refers to those who have a disease test positive or true positive rate, and *specificity* refers to those who do not have the disease, test negative, or the true negative rate.

CHAPTER 2: THE PRESCRIBER'S ROLE

1. **a.** Exceptions include circumstances in which serious harm or death is likely to occur without the intervention, and during an emergency circumstance when the patient is incapable of providing consent and a surrogate is not available to provide the consent.
2. **b.** Negotiation is not part of informed consent.
3. **d.** Clinicians should use plain language, provide education about their illness, explain potential benefits and risks of medication, and alternative options if available.
4. **a.** Respect and autonomy.
5. **d.** All of the above are correct.

CHAPTER 3: THE BRAIN AND NERVOUS SYSTEM

1. **c.** *Pharmacodynamics* is the study of a drug's molecular, biochemical, and physiologic effects or actions on the body.
2. **a.** A partial agonist can produce an effect within a cell that is not maximal and then block the receptor to a full agonist.

3. **b.** *Affinity* is a term that refers to the drug property that describes its unique ability to bind to the target receptors.
4. **a.** The process described is known as *neuroplasticity* or *neural plasticity* (brain plasticity). The human brain has a remarkable capacity to generate new neuronal connections, adapt, and change throughout the life span to enhance daily functioning.
5. **c.** An *excitatory neurotransmitter* triggers an electrical signal that is transmitted down the cell to activate the receiving neuron.

CHAPTER 4: NEUROTRANSMITTERS OVERVIEW

1. **c.** Drugs that increase acetylcholine levels in the brain are used in patients with Alzheimer's disease.
2. **d.** Nicotinic receptors on acetylcholine are also located in the brain's reward pathway and are hypothesized to underlie nicotine's addictive properties.
3. **a.** Glutamate is the major mediator of excitatory signals in neurotransmission.
4. **a.** GABA also plays an important role in behavior and cognition, such as impulsivity and risky decision-making.
5. **a.** Mu opioid receptors are linked to mood, pain, and reward.

CHAPTER 5: ANTIDEPRESSANTS

1. **a.** Tricyclic antidepressants are to be used with caution due to inducing a blockade of alpha-1 adrenergic receptors (dizziness or hypotension), their anticholinergic and sedating side effects, and narrow therapeutic index.
2. **c.** There are three SSRIs that are FDA approved for children: fluoxetine, escitalopram, and bupropion.
3. **a.** Risk of recurrence and persistent symptoms
4. **c.** Thyroid-stimulating hormone.
5. **c.** Fluoxetine

CHAPTER 6: ANXIOLYTICS AND ANTIANXIETY MEDICATIONS

1. **d.** Psychotherapy is the first-line therapy for children and adolescents with anxiety.
2. **d.** Risks associated with benzodiazepines include dependence, somnolence, and tolerance.
3. **d.** Nonbenzodiazepine anxiolytics include propranolol, gabapentin, and buspirone.
4. **b.** Catapres is not FDA approved for anxiety disorders in children or adults.
5. **a.** Glutamate is an excitatory neurotransmitter, and GABA is inhibitory.

CHAPTER 7: ANTIPSYCHOTIC MEDICATIONS

1. **a.** To begin administering clozaril, a minimum ANC value at baseline of 1,500/uL is required for the general population and a minimum of 1,000/uL for individuals with benign ethnic neutropenia.
2. **c.** Antipsychotics should be used with caution in older adults due to their potential to trigger inappropriate antidiuretic hormone secretion (SIADH), cause hyponatremia, increase stroke risk, increase rate of cognitive decline, and increase mortality.
3. **a.** The main difference between SGAs (or atypical antipsychotics) and FGAs (or typical antipsychotics) is that SGAs have dopaminergic- and serotonergic-blocking properties.
4. **b.** Tardive dyskinesia is a neurologic disorder characterized by involuntary movements, such as tongue protrusion, side-to-side movement of the jaw, lip smacking, puckering and pursing, and rapid eye blinking, as well as movements of the arms, legs, and trunk, and is a side effect associated with antipsychotic medications.
5. **a.** Treatment for EPS includes prescribing benztropin (Cogentin), lowering medication dosage, and discontinuing or changing medication. Dantrolene is used in the treatment of neuroleptic malignant syndrome (NMS).

CHAPTER 8: MOOD STABILIZERS

1. **c.** A baseline blood urea nitrogen, creatinine, electrolytes, thyroid function, and electrocardiogram are required before starting lithium. A CT scan is not required to start lithium.
2. **a.** Have a first-degree relative with bipolar disorder
3. **a.** Reliable and valid instruments can be used to detect the presence or absence of symptoms, help make a formal diagnosis, assess changes in symptom severity, and monitor client outcomes.
4. **a.** Anxiety, agitation, anger/irritability, attentional disturbance—distractibility
5. **b.** Due to cyclothymia's insidious onset and timing of onset, it can also be hard to tell whether mood symptoms are normal ups and downs, since youths are prone to hormonal fluctuations, labile mood, and overreacting to minor stressors and disappointments, or if these are signs of a mental health condition.

CHAPTER 9: STIMULANTS/NEURODEVELOPMENTAL DISORDERS

1. **d.** All of the above warrant a referral to a specialist.
2. **a.** The prefrontal cortex (PFC)
3. **d.** It has been absolutely determined that ADHD risk factors include excessive sugar intake, excessive television viewing, or poor parenting management.

4. **b.** There is no single test to diagnose ADHD; therefore, gathering information from multiple sources, which can include ADHD symptom checklists, standardized behavior rating scales, a detailed history of past and current functioning, and information obtained from collateral sources, is warranted.
5. **c.** Stuttering is not a symptom of ADHD.

CHAPTER 10: ANTIDEMENTIA

1. **a.** Changes in acetylcholine synthesis
2. **c.** Memantine is an acetylcholinesterase inhibitor.
3. **d.** All of the above help with medication compliance.
4. **b.** Vascular dementia is the second most common form of dementia after Alzheimer's disease. It's caused when decreased blood flow damages brain tissue.
5. **b.** Increased air pollution and having a first-degree relative with AD

CHAPTER 11: SLEEP DISORDERS

1. **b.** Dreaming occurs during the rapid eye movement sleep stage.
2. **a.** During periods of darkness, the pineal gland located in the brain helps to regulate circadian rhythms and releases the hormone melatonin.
3. **c.** Cognitive behavioral therapy for insomnia is the first-line treatment and the gold standard intervention in the management of insomnia.
4. **d.** This statement is false. In older adults, use of benzodiazepines does not need to be avoided in the treatment of insomnia if they are prescribed in low doses.
5. **c.** Treatment goals in the management of insomnia include the improvement of sleep quality, sleep duration, and sleep satisfaction, and reducing daytime impairments caused by excessive daytime sleepiness.

CHAPTER 12: NONMEDICATION TREATMENTS

1. **a.** Caffeine inhibits CYP450 1A2 and increases clozapine levels.
2. **d.** Grapefruit juice *inhibits* the CYP450 3A4 isoforms due to bioflavonoids that *raise* bioavailability concentrations of psychotropic drugs.
3. **a.** SMART is an acronym for specific, measurable, attainable, relevant, and timely goals for personal improvement. SMART goals help clients track their progress and alter their plans when necessary.
4. **a.** Psychoeducation provides the client, family, and/or caregivers with information about the illness; its course, causes, treatment, prognosis, and available supportive resources; and allows the clinician to respond to questions or concerns.

5. **c.** It is important to inquire about caffeine intake at each follow-up visit because caffeine alters the dissolution profile of psychotropic medications, alters gastrointestinal pH, affects gastrointestinal emptying times, and impacts the formation of inhibiting glucose-6-phosphatase that can impact medication levels.

Index

www.ingramcontent.com/pod-product-compliance
Ingram Content Group UK Ltd.
Pitfield, Milton Keynes, MK11 3LW, UK
UKHW021353110926
15107UKWH00004B/8

9 780826 184535

OTHER *ESSENTIALS* BOOKS

Essentials on **ADOLESCENT HEALTH FOR NURSING AND HEALTH PROFESSIONALS**: A Care Guide (*Herrman*)

Essentials for the **ADULT-GERONTOLOGY ACUTE CARE NURSE PRACTITIONER** (*Carpenter*)

Essentials for the **ANTEPARTUM AND POSTPARTUM NURSE**: A Nursing Orientation and Care Guide (*Davidson*)

Essentials Workbook for **CARDIAC DYSRHYTHMIAS AND 12-LEAD EKGs** (*Desmarais*)

Essentials for the **CARDIAC SURGERY NURSE**: Caring for Cardiac Surgery Patients, Third Edition (*Hodge*)

Essentials for **CAREER SUCCESS IN NURSING**: Making the Most of Mentoring (*Vance*)

Essentials for the **CATH LAB NURSE**, Second Edition (*McCulloch*)

Essentials for the **CLASSROOM NURSING INSTRUCTOR**: Classroom Teaching (*Yoder-Wise, Kowalski*)

Essentials for the **CLINICAL NURSE LEADER** (*Wilcox, Deerhake*)

Essentials for the **CLINICAL NURSE MANAGER**: Managing a Changing Workplace, Second Edition (*Fry*)

Essentials for the **CLINICAL NURSING INSTRUCTOR**: Clinical Teaching, Third Edition (*Kan, Stabler-Haas*)

Essentials on **COMBATING NURSE BULLYING, INCIVILITY, AND WORKPLACE VIOLENCE**: What Nurses Need to Know (*Ciocco*)

Essentials About **COMPETENCY-BASED EDUCATION IN NURSING**: How to Teach Competency Mastery (*Wittmann-Price, Gittings*)

Essentials for the **CRITICAL CARE NURSE**, Second Edition (*Hewett*)

Essentials About **CURRICULUM DEVELOPMENT IN NURSING**: How to Develop and Evaluate Educational Programs, Second Edition (*McCoy, Anema*)

Essentials for **DEMENTIA CARE**: What Nurses Need to Know, Second Edition (*Miller*)

Essentials for **DEVELOPING A NURSING ACADEMIC PORTFOLIO**: What You Really Need to Know (*Wittmann-Price*)

Essentials About **DIVERSITY, EQUITY, AND INCLUSION IN NURSING**: Building Competencies for an Antiracism Practice (*Davis*)

Essentials for **DNP ROLE DEVELOPMENT**: A Career Navigation Guide (*Menonna-Quinn, Tortorella Genova*)

Essentials About **EKGs FOR NURSES**: The Rules of Identifying EKGs (*Landrum*)

Essentials for the **ER NURSE**: Guide to a Successful Emergency Department Orientation, Fourth Edition (*Buettner*)

Essentials for **EVIDENCE-BASED PRACTICE IN NURSING**: Third Edition (*Godshall*)

Essentials for the **FAITH COMMUNITY NURSE**: Implementing FCN/Parish Nursing (*Hickman*)

Essentials About **FORENSIC NURSING**: What You Need to Know (*Scannell*)

Essentials on **GENETICS AND GENOMICS FOR NURSES**: Practical Applications (*Subasic*)

Essentials for the **GERONTOLOGY NURSE**: A Nursing Care Guide (*Eliopoulos*)

Essentials About **GI AND LIVER DISEASES FOR NURSES**: What APRNs Need to Know (*Chaney*)

Essentials About the **GYNECOLOGICAL EXAM**: A Professional Guide for NPs, PAs, and Midwives, Second Edition (*Secor, Fantasia*)

Essentials in **HEALTH INFORMATICS FOR NURSES** (*Hardy*)

Essentials for **HEALTH PROMOTION IN NURSING**: Promoting Wellness (*Miller*)

Essentials for Nurses About **HOME IN FUSION THERAPY**: The Expert's Best Practice Guide (*Gorski*)

Essentials for the **HOSPICE NURSE**: A Concise Guide to End-of-Life Care, Second Edition (*Wright*)

Essentials about **LGBTQ+ CARE FOR NURSES** (*Traister*)

Essentials for the **LONG-TERM CARE NURSE**: What Nursing Home and Assisted Living Nurses Need to Know (*Eliopoulos*)

Essentials to **LOVING YOUR RESEARCH PROJECT**: A Stress-Free Guide for Novice Researchers in Nursing and Healthcare (*Marshall*)

Essentials for **MAKING THE MOST OF YOUR CAREER IN NURSING** (*Redulla*)

Essentials for **MANAGING PATIENTS WITH A PSYCHIATRIC DISORDER**: What RNs, NPs, and New Psych Nurses Need to Know (*Marshall*)

Essentials About **MEDICAL CANNABIS AND OPIOIDS**: Minimizing Opioid Use Through Cannabis (*Smith, Smith*)

Essentials for the **MEDICAL OFFICE NURSE**: What You Really Need to Know (*Richmeier*)

Essentials for the **MEDICAL–SURGICAL NURSE**: Clinical Orientation (*Ciocco*)

Essentials for **MIDWIVES**: Labor & Delivery Orientation, Third Edition (*Groll*)

Essentials for the **OPERATING ROOM NURSE**, Third Edition (*Criscitelli*)

Essentials for **PATIENT SAFETY IN NURSING**: How to Decrease Medical Errors and Improve Patient Outcomes (*Hunt*)

Essentials for **PSYCHOPHARMACOLOGY FOR NURSE PRACTITIONERS** (*Goldin*)